IF YOUR CLOSET COULD TALK, WHAT WOULD IT SAY ABOUT YOU?

"She's got clothes in here she's never even worn—
with the price tags still attached!"

"That fuchsia suede miniskirt was an impulse buy—
why won't she let it go, already?"

"Pssst—she hasn't fit into those jeans since the Clinton administration. . . ."

"Can't she see that buying one pair of navy pants
would give those print blouses a whole new life?"

Let's face it: our closets are finite spaces, while our clothing and accessories could have their own galaxy! So why do so many of them just hang there, unused?

Whether you love to shop for clothes or hate it, follow fashion trends or your own beat, you can now make order out of closet chaos. Much more than just an organizing guide, *"I DON'T HAVE A THING TO WEAR"* gets to the heart of your clothing issues—from "emotional" shopping, to wardrobe blind spots, to "someday" thinking. You'll learn how to build a wardrobe, how to keep your wardrobe working for you when you move to a more or less formal workplace, or to another part of the country, and even when you gain or lose weight.

Here are the guidelines you need to shop wisely, organize easily, and create a wardrobe that makes you feel attractive, comfortable, powerful, sexy, and completely yourself—every day!

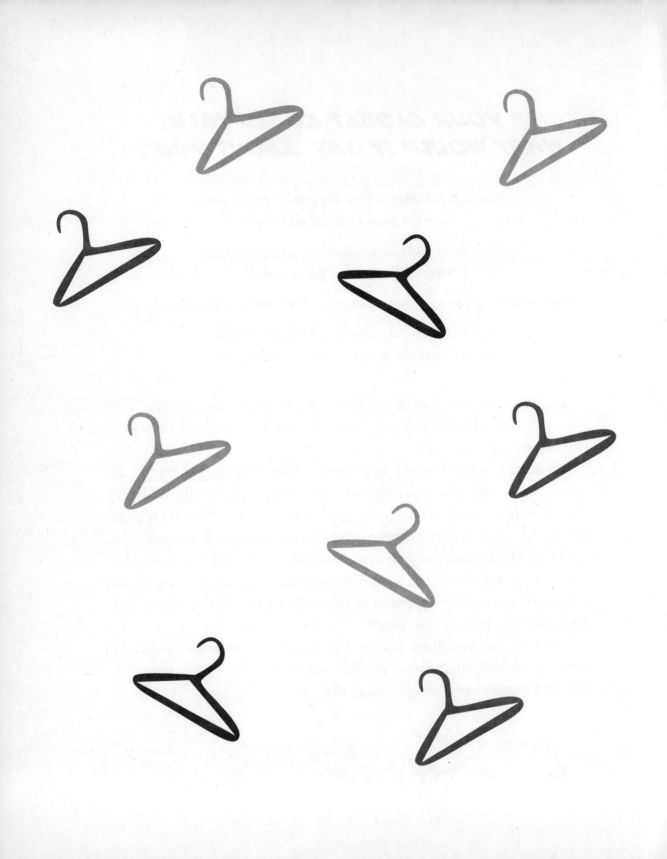

"I DON'T HAVE A THING TO WEAR"

THE PSYCHOLOGY OF YOUR CLOSET

JUDIE TAGGART

AND

JACKIE WALKER,
THE "DR. OF CLOSETOLOGY"

POCKET BOOKS
New York London Toronto Sydney Singapore

POCKET BOOKS, a division of Simon & Schuster, Inc.
1230 Avenue of the Americas, New York, NY 10020

ISBN: 0-7434-6644-6

First Pocket Books trade paperback edition August 2003

10   9   8   7   6   5   4   3   2

POCKET and colophon are registered trademarks of
Simon & Schuster, Inc.

Designed by Jaime Putorti

Manufactured in the United States of America

For information regarding special discounts for bulk purchases,
please contact Simon & Schuster Special Sales at 1-800-456-6798
or business@simonandschuster.com

To John, Shara and Jennifer, with love and affection.

Judie

To the three men in my life: Neil, Brian, and Mark, for always being there for me with encouragement, enthusiasm, and love.

Jackie

ACKNOWLEDGMENTS

Our sincere thanks to our agents Stedman Mays and Mary Tahan for understanding, steadfast encouragement and diplomacy in guiding us while maintaining their unfailing sense of humor; to Micki Nuding, our style-wise editor, for her insight into our message, editorial expertise, and keen wit; and to Sherry Hutchinson, our marvelous illustrator, for effortlessly tuning in to our frequency.

Judie wishes to thank:

Bill Blass, Ralph Lauren, and all the designers and fashionistas I've met, interviewed, and profiled who shaped my taste and propelled my career both in merchandising and as fashion editor of *The Tampa Tribune;* to Jay Stein, Jack Williams, and Mike Fisher at Stein Mart for entrusting me to represent your company and meet hundreds of women in twenty-eight states, many of whom became members of the store's Boutique Program of community advisers. These engaged, accomplished, and involved women are on every page. And last, thank you Jackie for your unfailing optimism, support, erudite knowledge about human resources, and friendship.

Jackie wishes to acknowledge and thank:

The many mentors who have come into my life with words of inspiration and wisdom, beginning with my parents, for dressing me beautifully on the inside and challenging me on the outside; Andy and Irene Katz, for wise business advice and friendship; Sharon Kummelman, for being a sea of calm; to Burdine's, for taking me from the fashion area to human resources—a true learning experience and the first step toward developing my company, Option Dressing; to Beverly Martin, for the opportunity to be the national spokesperson for women's conferencing for JCPenney, exposing me to female groups and helping me shape my philosophies. To Judie, my writing partner, for taking this journey with me. I treasure all of the moments and appreciate everything you have taught me. Finally, to all the women I have worked for and with, you have given me great joy, fun, and knowledge.

In closing—we extend special thanks to J. Kevin Thompson, Ph.D., a psychology professor, and Dore Beach, Ph.D., a psychology counselor, both of the University of South Florida, and to Johannes A. G. Rhodin, M.D., Ph.D., USF Medical College, for sharing your professional knowledge, research, and counsel.

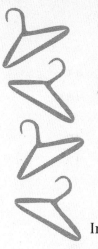

CONTENTS

Introduction   xv

CHAPTER ONE
THE CIRCLE OF YOUR LIFE—
FAMILY, BUSINESS, FUN, AND ROMANCE   1
  The Circle of Your Life Game   3
  Why You Have Nothing to Wear   6
  Someday Clothes   9
  Changes and Transitions   10
  The Pitfalls of Poor Shopping Habits   12
  Clone Dressing   13
  Create a Clothes Diary   15
  Your Plan   17

CHAPTER TWO
LET'S DEFINE YOU   19
  Self-Discovery Quiz   19
  Self-Knowledge Is the Key   31
  Transitions and Personal Growth   32
  Esteem Issues—Getting to the Heart of the Matter   34
  Age Isn't What It Used to Be   36
  Attitude, Interests, and Psychographics   37
  Finances and the Size of Your Closet   39

CHAPTER THREE

THE PSYCHOLOGY OF YOUR CLOSET   43

     A Daily Search for Self-Esteem   44

     Secrets and Revelations   45

     Truthfully—What Percentage of Your Clothes Do You Wear?   47

     The Mirror and Insecurities   47

     How Your Past Poisoned Your Well of Confidence   51

     Flashbacks Can Set You Free   54

     Unveiling the Real You in Your Closet   56

     Your History Is Not Who You Are Today   58

CHAPTER FOUR

DISCOVER YOUR FASHION PERSONA—

INTERNAL SELF-EXPRESSION   59

     The Seven Dominant Fashion Personalities   60

         1. The Classic—Timeless and Conservative   61

         2. The Natural—Direct, Unpretentious, Low-Maintenance   63

         3. The Modernist—Updated, Sleek, Sophisticated   64

         4. The Romantic—Traditional, Nostalgic, Ladylike   67

         5. Fashion Trend Tracker—on the Cutting Edge   69

         6. Mood Dresser—Bohemian, Creative, Artistic   71

         7. Dramatic Women—Ready for Their Close-up   74

     A Caution   78

     The Role of Fashion Trends in Persona   79

     The Bell Curve of Fashion Trends   80

     Discovering Your Fashion Persona   82

CHAPTER FIVE

CLOSETOLOGY 101:

A BLUEPRINT TO CLEAR THE CHAOS AND ESTABLISH ORDER   91

     Fear, Potential, and the Memories in Your Closet   94

     Closet Insight Quiz   96

Getting in the Mind-set   97

Separation Anxiety   98

Someday Clothes, Your Nostalgia Corner, Markdown
   Mistakes, and Others   99

The Organization Blueprint   100

Accessories Organization   103

The Payoff!   106

Tips and Tricks for Setting Up Your Closet   107

CHAPTER SIX

PROPORTION POLITICS: HORIZONTAL LINE DRESSING   109

Comfort Boxes and What They Mean to You   113

Moving the Lines to Create Your Most Flattering
   Visual Impression   116

Say Yes, Say No   131

CHAPTER SEVEN

BUILDING A WARDROBE FROM THE BOTTOMS UP   133

Learning How to Dress from the Bottoms Up   138

Bottom Basics—Pants, Jeans, Shorts   139

Skirts—the Right Style for You   143

Learn While Pretending You Are a Buyer   146

Visit the Mall—a Homework Assignment   148

What You Learn in Your Own Closet   149

CHAPTER EIGHT

THE HIGH SIDE OF BUSINESS CASUAL   151

From the Trenches of Training Seminars   153

It's a Slight Relaxation, Not a Pajama Party   154

A New Way of Thinking   156

A Business Casual System That Works   158

The Final Analysis   161

CHAPTER NINE
LET'S GO SHOPPING!   **165**
   The "I Hate to Shop" Epidemic   167
   Attacking Dysfunctional Shopping Emporiums   169
   Size Wise Savvy   173
   True Tales of Sale-Rack Philosophy and Success   174
   Sale Tips: Making Every Dollar Count   176
   Seasonal Fashion Calendar   177
   Return Policies   178
   Six Keys to Becoming a Laser Shopper   180
   Travel Stops and Trend Reruns   180
   Cruising Catalogs and Shopping on the Internet:
      Hazards and Benefits   181
   Let's Go Shopping—a Quiz for You   183

CHAPTER TEN
PUNCH PIECES AND FINISHING TOUCHES   **187**
   Why You Choose and Wear Them   188
   Jewelry Tells the World about You   192
   Size and Symmetry   194
   Self-Expression in a Handbag   198
   Kicking Up Your Heels   203
   Belts: The Middle Ground   206
   Glasses Project Attitude and Charisma   207
   Accessories Entice and Add Focus   208

CHAPTER ELEVEN
TRAVELING: YOUR SUITCASE AS YOUR CLOSET   **211**
   The Most Common Mistakes   213
   A Master Plan   215
   The Five *Ws* of Suitcase Simplification   216
   Do Your Weight Lifting at the Gym   217

Starting with the Basics   217
A Packing Pyramid   220
Do a Dress Rehearsal   222
What Goes Where?   223
Color Plans   225
Pivotal Pieces Add Versatility   226
Packing Tips   228

Fifty Bonus Hot Tips   231
  Insider Secrets You Need to Know   231
Index   239

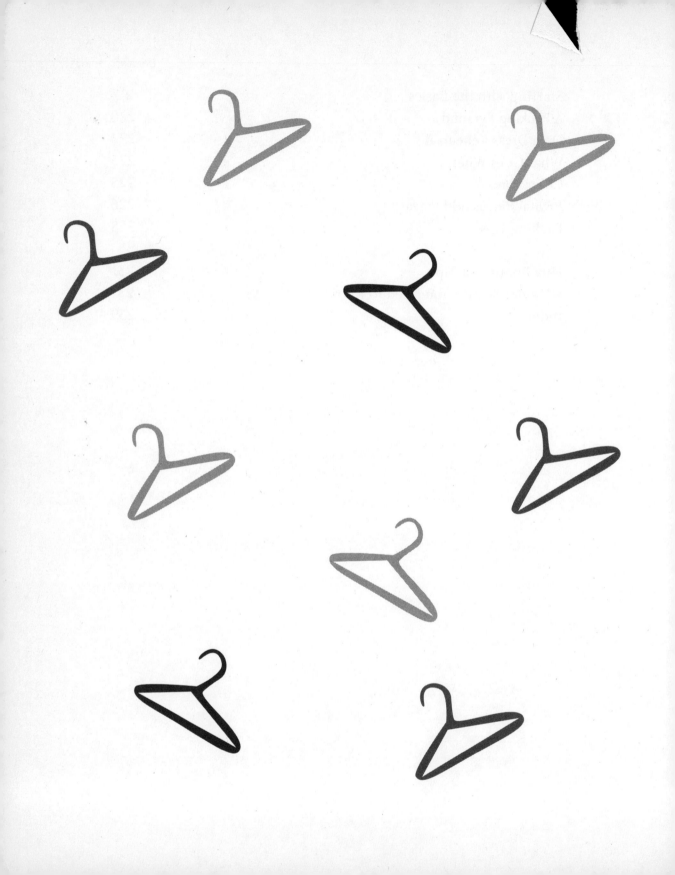

INTRODUCTION

While traveling the nation meeting hundreds of women, the one phrase we heard over and over again is, "I don't have a thing to wear." We asked, "Why?" No one knew. This statement was an emotional response, not a fashion dilemma, because the women often admitted their closets were full of clothes. We discovered that each closet represented a collection of their life experiences, attitudes, fears, ambitions, and hopes for the future. How you present yourself is deeply ingrained in your psyche. Clothes serve as props to build your image and self-esteem. Each item you select for your wardrobe is an emotionally driven extension of yourself. Dressing yourself starts inside, not on the surface.

Each chapter of our book encourages you to examine your motives, instincts, selections, and behavior patterns when selecting your clothing. In learning about the psychology of your closet and how you dress from the inside out, you will not only discover more about yourself, but also be enlightened about women around you: friends, fellow business associates, and family.

Certain sections of the book will resonate more deeply with you, resulting in moments of self-revelation you will find surprising and insightful. You may experience a change in perception, gain more self-confidence through self-knowledge, and find a touch of adventure and challenge teasing you to try to become more than you are now and what deep in your heart you authentically hope to be.

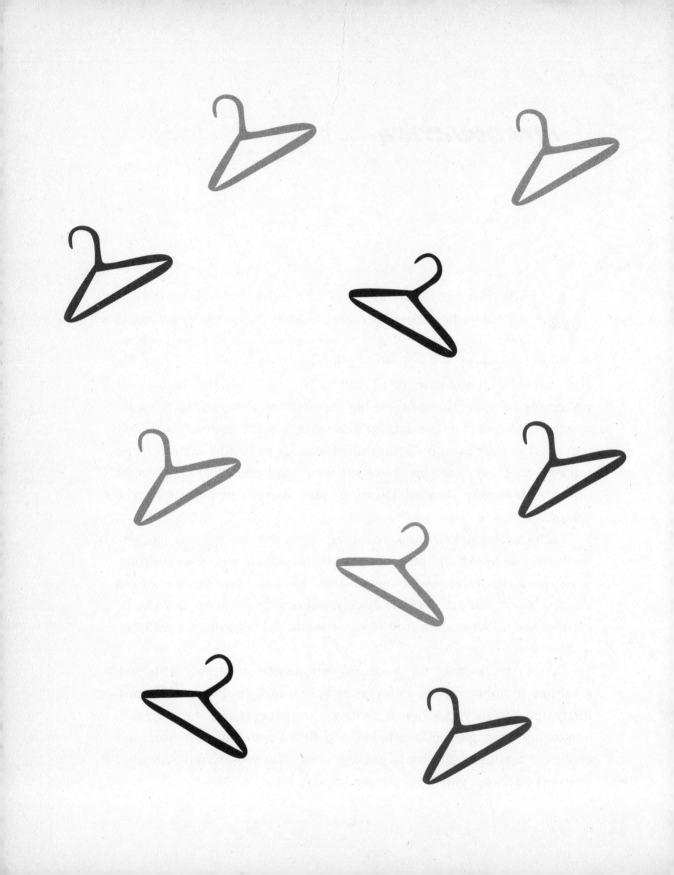

CHAPTER ONE

THE CIRCLE OF YOUR LIFE—FAMILY, BUSINESS, FUN, AND ROMANCE

Fantasy and romance play a huge role in fashion. I have seen women buy clothes and say, "This will be wonderful to wear to Ascot," even though the chances of their going to Ascot that season are very, very slim. It has to do with fantasy.

BILL BLASS, DESIGNER

The scene is all too familiar. It's 8 A.M. and Kay is running late. She has an important meeting and luncheon today. She is in front of her mirror, pulling on one thing, trying another, rejecting as she goes, delving deeper and deeper into her closet as she searches for the elusive ideal ensemble. Now she is tugging a hopelessly snug olive green skirt over her hips. Forget it. Next comes the cranberry pantsuit—too much, too loud. The green gabardine suit worked a long time ago, but where is the blouse that goes with it? The gray pants are too short. (She'd promised herself she would get them altered.) The new paisley blouse is gorgeous, but it doesn't work with either the gray or green pants. (Come to think of it, it never seems to work with anything.) Kay presses on.

Jumbled among these seemingly unworkable work clothes are several colorful ski sweaters. She passes the ski pants and several colors of lightweight fleece turtlenecks, remembering that she never went skiing once this season, and in fact has rarely gone since she decided to learn three years ago.

Kay impatiently pushes aside three beautiful cocktail gowns in her effort to find her trusty brown blazer. Where *is* that thing? Oh, no! It's at the cleaners. She avoided taking it there as long as she could, fearing a

• 1 •

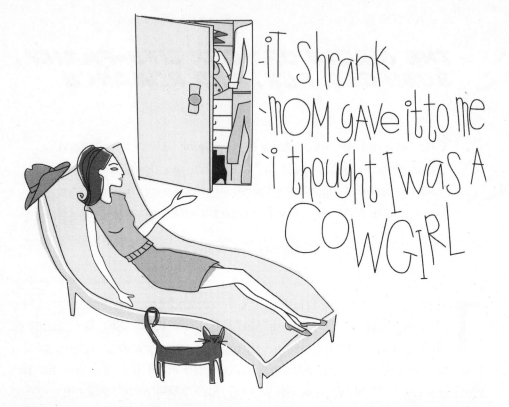

-iT Shrank
-mOm gave it to me
-i thought I was A
COWGIRL

morning exactly like this one—when nothing else would please her and she needed to turn to that staunch dependable. Now, at this critical moment, it is missing in action. Maybe the dotted skirt and black jacket will work with a white shell blouse? No, that's too summery. Okay, how about the brown pants and blouse with a muted plaid jacket? Yikes! She just wore that Monday.

Two more skirts are way too tight. In fact, they've been too tight for a couple of years now. Wasn't she going to buy another black skirt? Hmmm. That was the day she bought the beaded evening bag instead. Which, come to think of it, she's never had occasion to carry. It's stunning, though.

Well, what's it to be? Looks like the black wool crepe suit with a black turtleneck. Again. Kay has exhausted herself trying to put together an outfit that gives her the right click of confidence. Surrounded by heaps of discarded clothes on her chair, bed, and floor, the thought once again crosses Kay's mind: *I don't have a thing to wear!*

Does any of this sound familiar? Have you ever found yourself in a similar scenario? So have we, and so has every one of our clients. But guess what? There's a simple reason why. Get ready to discover the answer by playing the "Circle of Your Life" Game.

A simple circle is the key to solving the age-old mystery of why women have closets full of clothes but nothing to wear. The Circle of Your Life Game is the first step in getting your wardrobe in sync with your life, and ladies, it's no exaggeration when we say that this exercise is a life-altering experience. Time and again, when we go through this exercise with our clients, they are stunned. They come away enlightened and inspired, and they certainly never look at their wardrobes in the same way again. Here's how it works.

THE CIRCLE OF YOUR LIFE GAME

You are going to create the Circle of Your Life. This is the first step to finding the real you in your closet. The goal is for you to discover exactly what parts of your wardrobe are missing. Your Circle of Life also enables you to make a shopping list and helps you to understand why your closet needs to be in harmony with your life.

The game takes about one hour, so plan to concentrate, and get ready to find out more about yourself "sartorially speaking" than you ever dreamed. Okay? Here we go!

STEP 1. On a blank piece of paper (we recommend 8½-by-11-inch), draw a circle. You are going to create a pie chart, a simple circle divided into slices of various sizes. The size of each portion is based on your life's activities.

STEP 2. On a second sheet of paper, list every category of activity you perform (clothed!) in your waking moments. These activities should be comprehensive—evening, weekend, seasonal, and even occasional activities go on this list, along with those you engage in every day.

STEP 3. Estimate the percentage of time you spend on each activity. To get a true picture, base your circle on a four-week period, about one month. We find using a month as a guide gives people a broader sense of how they spend their time, as weekend diversions may vary.

For instance, suppose your average waking day runs from 7 A.M. to 11 P.M.

7 A.M. to 11 P.M. = 16 hours

16 hours x 7 days = 112 hours in a week

112 hours in a week x 4 weeks = 448 hours per month

Now, figure out the hours you spend on each activity in a four-week period. Then use this figure to calculate the percentage of time you spend on that activity. For instance, if you work forty hours a week, you work 160 hours in four weeks. Divide 160 hours by 448 monthly hours: you work 36 percent of your circle. Suppose your social life totals forty-six hours in a month. Divide forty-six hours by 448, and the percentage is 10 percent for social life. If you have children, your activities with them may take, say, forty-two hours a week, or 168 hours. Divide 168 hours by 448 hours, and your percentage is 38. Estimate your activities and percentages until your circle represents 100 percent of your life. Write these percentages next to the activities listed on your paper. You may need to further subdivide these percentages after you have completed your circle.

STEP 4. Returning to your circle, divide it into slices according to the percentages you have just created.

STEP 5. Within each slice of your pie, list a life activity. Next to the circle, list the types of clothing you wear to perform this life activity. For your work slice, write what you wear to work. For some women this means corporate suits, trousers, twin sweater sets, and knit layering pieces, while for others it may mean a more business casual mix, such as khakis and sweaters, with dresses, skirts, and suits only occasionally.

NOTE: If your work tends to neatly divide itself into casual and more formal corporate dressing (for instance, if you are a consultant who works at home in jeans 60 percent of the time and dons designer suits for meetings with clients the remaining 40 percent), you might want to subdivide your work pie slice accordingly. With the changing rules about workplace dressing and the millions of people now working out of their homes and in flexible work situations, the individual variations on work dressing requirements are endless. That's why we have devoted an entire chapter to the nuances of business casual dressing.

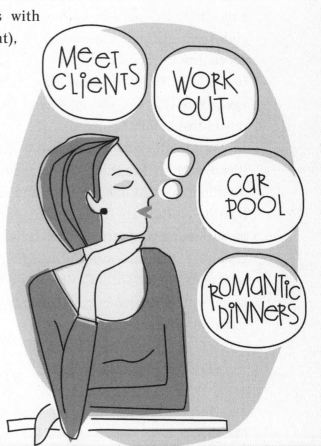

If you work at home and commute electronically, list that percentage and what you usually wear to work at home. If you dress in business clothes to work at home, put that down. Many people do so to mentally get in the groove of working. We know men and women who get up, get dressed in a suit, walk to their office at the other end of the house, and take their jacket off. On the other hand, many businesspeople working in their homes plop down in front of the computer in jeans, slouchy cotton knits, or pajamas. If that is you, put it down.

And speaking of pajamas, if you come home from work and immediately change into loungewear or jammies, we would categorize that as casual. Sleepwear to us is a different thing.

Next, list your clothing choices for your other waking activities in the appropriate pie slices. You might wear similar things while doing various family duties, such as grocery shopping, carpooling, and volunteering, so write those in one slice of your chart. You may need dressier things for club meetings and luncheons. Working out may mean leggings and a sports bra for aerobics classes, but khaki shorts and tees for your daily two-mile walks. Write those down in separate slices and assign percentages. Here is where you may need to divide your percentages further to reflect this breakdown.

On the other hand, feel free to cluster types of clothes. For example, if you wear similar things to go antiquing and attending club meetings, list them both in one pie slice and determine a percentage. Beach and boating clothes are often similar and could share a slice. If socializing means going with friends or colleagues straight from work and not changing your business clothes, you should note this under your business clothing pie slice. Clothing you wear when entertaining at home or going out with friends on weekends may be the same and can be combined in a slice.

WHY YOU HAVE NOTHING TO WEAR

Now for the moment of truth. Your circle chart should look something like this:

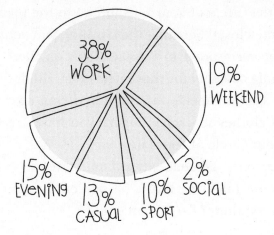

38%
WORK

19%
WEEKEND

15%
EVENING

13%
CASUAL

10%
SPORT

2%
SOCIAL

YOUR CHART

Work 38%
Suits, jackets, tops, pants, pantsuits
Exercise/sports 10%
Golf/tennis/aerobics/jogging
Evenings out 15%
Dresses, separates, long skirts
Social 2%
Evening gown, cocktail dresses, and dressy suits
At home casual 13%
Jeans, knit pants and big tops, shorts, shifts
Weekends 19%
Dressy casual tops, pants, skirts, tees

Now take the Circle of Your Life and go to the place where you start each day . . . the closet! Separate the clothing you actually wear into the categories that correspond to the pie slices on the Circle of Your Life. Create a separate category for those items that either don't fit into one of your categories, or are items you cannot or do not wear. Now compare the percentage of clothes in each category you have created with the percentages on your Circle of Your Life chart.

We guarantee the percentages will not match.

You may work full-time, but is 38 percent of your closet ready and willing to take you there? Do 20 percent of your clothes meet the needs you have for leisure activities? And why does that pile of unworn items represent 30 percent of your closet?

Diagnosis: your closet is not in harmony with your life.

"A simple circle is the key to solving the age-old mystery of why women have closets full of clothes and nothing to wear."

We often inquire, "What percentage of the clothes in your closet do you actually wear?" The answer: 20 percent to 40 percent—at best. If you wear only 20 to 40 percent of what is in your closet, how can you dress 100 percent of your life?

Let's take the case of Kay, a working mother with two small children, whom we met at the beginning of this chapter. She is a real-life client of ours. When Kay completed the Circle of Your Life activity, she was shocked by the results. Although she had started out thinking she had plenty to wear to work (35 percent of her pie), after she separated out the work clothes she never wore, she was left with only a few basic pieces. Kay realized that in an effort to vary the blacks and browns and neutral tones she preferred, she had been purchasing bright colors and prints that she never wore once she got them home—they just didn't feel right.

She found also that although she wore her leisure/kid time jeans and tee shirts over and over, she never felt good in them. Yet when she shopped, she spent no time or effort on acquiring casual pieces that made her look and feel good, despite needing to wear these clothes every day. Kay also learned she was a bit of a dreamer, refusing to get rid of outfits and pieces she wore ten pounds ago but that hadn't looked good on her for years. Ditto her unrealistic attitude concerning sportswear: lots of beautiful ski clothes, but no skiing! And yet, once again, why did she make no effort to find flattering jeans and chic tops and sweaters for the many day-to-day activities she needed them for? Finally, Kay got an eye-opener about her shopping habits—lots of glamorous, often-expensive pieces that played no role even on her occasional evenings out with her husband or friends. Why was Kay making these same mistakes over and over?

Whether we realize it or not, many of us make the same mistakes again and again in our own closets. Once you understand why you are not creating a wardrobe in sync with the Circle of Your Life, you can start working on how to fix the problem.

SOMEDAY CLOTHES

Does the Circle of Your Life reflect a nonexistent social life? No black-tie balls or spiffy cocktail parties and dinners? Then why are those three beaded and sequined dresses with markdown tags hanging in your closet? Or maybe your Circle reflects no time for exercise, yet there are those flashy workout clothes, hiking boots, and jogging clothes, or lots of impractical ski wear.

These are your "Someday Clothes." Someday Clothes are expressions of intentions that have not materialized. *Someday I will join the gym. Someday I will get back to my social life.* Why is your closet filled with clothes to dress for what you never do, and missing the clothes you need for who you really are? Remember, your activities dictate your wardrobe needs. This principle is a key to "closet harmony."

Are we saying that women shouldn't have goals to improve their appearance or their lifestyle? Should Kay abandon forever her desire to lose a few pounds? Do we advise her to let go of all efforts to ski as an unrealistic daydream? Of course not! We encourage every client we talk with to strive to be the best that she can be. But, ladies, we encourage you first to streamline, update, expand, weed out, and improve your closet *for the body, comfort level, tastes, preferences, self-image, lifestyle, and Circle of Your Life you have now.*

CHANGES AND TRANSITIONS

Often a woman sabotages herself by failing to recognize life transitions that affect her clothing needs. Transitions mean that you may need new clothes. Here are some examples of "out-of-balance" closets. See if you identify with any of these real-life situations.

Weight Changes

Susan is a real estate agent. In the last year she gained fifteen pounds due to stress and a new medication. Like Kay, very little in Susan's closet fits anymore. Each day she looks in her closet and becomes depressed. She works seven days a week, yet only 10 percent of her clothes are available to her. Is it any wonder her friend Linda comments, "I love that dress! I love it every time you wear it." Neither Susan nor Kay wants to give up forever the goal of losing some weight. But neither one can afford to buy an entire new wardrobe in one fell swoop either. So what's the answer?

First, both Susan and Kay need to accept the reality—however temporary—of the numbers on their scale. By refusing to alter clothes or buy any standard pieces in a larger size (such as basic black pants, black skirt, etc.), they are condemning themselves to a daily ritual of misery when they go to get dressed. In chapter 5, we will look at realistic solutions for updating a wardrobe that no longer fits you without starting from scratch—and we'll give you a plan for taking those too-small "Someday Clothes" and selecting the best pieces to keep for when you reach your weight goals.

Job Changes

Barbara has just changed jobs—she's gone from a strict corporate environment to a business casual dress code. Everything in her closet feels stiff, stuffy, and too serious to wear when calling on her new clients. She doesn't have a lot of disposable income to go on a shopping spree (who does?), and she leaves the house every day feeling uncomfortable.

What do we tell clients like Barbara? *First, try to make use of what already exists.* Start with the pieces you have. Perhaps Barbara's corporate suits can be separated, and the jackets made to look more casual with khaki pants. Trousers and skirts can be relaxed with a twin sweater set. There are economical ways to make Barbara's Circle of Your Life work within her current closet. Chapter 5 will take a closer look at practical solutions to this very common situation too.

Geography Changes

Stella has been transferred from Orlando to San Francisco. In Florida, silk suits and bright colors slipped perfectly into her business wardrobe. Suddenly she is cold all the time—even in July and August—and everyone seems to be dressed in beige or black wool gabardine suits. It's easy to tell the tourists from the professionals in this City by the Bay. What a change from Orlando, where the casual lifestyle influenced everyone's wardrobe. Stella feels out of step and out of place.

New jobs and new locations often dictate changes in clothing patterns. Stella is not in Disney World anymore. San Francisco is a big city reeking with sophistication and filled with high-powered executives. She needs to sharpen her awareness of what clothing styles prevail in her new business culture. She'll need to rethink her entire wardrobe, starting with the purchase of a good all-weather coat plus three pieces—a blazer, skirt, and pants—in dark gray or black. Mixing her bright blouses with these dark basics will instantly start her wardrobe on a big-city track.

Life Transitions

Brittany just graduated from college. Four years of jeans and logo tee shirts made it a breeze to get dressed each day. Then came her dream job offer, an executive training position in New York City. She accepts, and while still in Tuscaloosa, she rushes out to purchase two suits, one navy and one gray. Two weeks into life in the Big Apple, Brittany stares into her closet in despair. She has nothing to wear. Already she is losing her fragile newfound sense of confidence and competence. Brittany should have planned her wardrobe search right along with her career search, analyzing the dress codes of the companies she met with during the interview process. This is a major change in life, and women facing such a transition will need to create a Circle of Your Life for their brand-new life, not for what they've been doing prior to this. Building a wardrobe takes time. Building a lifestyle wardrobe takes a plan.

A woman needs to rethink her wardrobe when she makes changes in herself, her career, and her lifestyle. Getting a new job, moving to a new city, getting married or divorced, or making any new, positive lifestyle choice means a woman may have to create a new Circle of Your Life for the new woman she is becoming.

THE PITFALLS OF POOR SHOPPING HABITS

Shopping habits may be your downfall in getting your closet in harmony with your life. Impulse purchases, super bargain buys, and Web catalog clicks may have set you off in the wrong direction more than once. In Kay's case, she tends to forget what her goals are when she enters a store—making glamorous impulse purchases such as a sequined bag is more fun than trying to find flattering casual pieces for the "mom" segment of her Circle of Your Life, or dealing with the need for a more updated dark suit for business meetings.

Right now, shopping is not about buying what she needs but about making herself feel good. In chapter 9, we'll show you how we helped Kay and dozens more of our clients find pleasure and satisfaction in working on real-life wardrobe goals when shopping.

"Your closet is not in harmony with your life."

Margo is a single mom. She works as a human resource executive in a major law firm. Her passion is bargain shopping, and she loads her closet with "steals" she cannot live without. She purchases for price, rather than desire for what she really wants or needs, then forgets to ever buy anything to match these orphan wardrobe pieces. Each day, her mornings are spent changing clothes at least a dozen times. Like thousands of us, Margo purchases out of emotion instead of using a plan. She lets her feelings take over, and she charges on without reason or thought. Before purchasing an impulse item, Margo needs to ask herself two questions: How many ways can I wear this? Will this fit into my Circle of Your Life? Margo desperately needs to create a Circle of Your Life and adjust her shopping habits accordingly. In chapter 9, we'll also learn how bargains and sales can help create the wardrobe you need instead of a closet full of unworn items.

CLONE DRESSING

Clone dressing can come over you so subtly you don't realize what's happening. It may strike because of your geographical location—in the

Southwest, broom skirts, western boots, and denim are considered wardrobe backbones. Or the people you work with or your crowd of friends may dictate it. Even the place you shop.

Cassie, a young mother on a tight budget, discovers a little shop specializing in crinkle rayon separates and long casual dresses. After her first $200 in purchases, the store offered her a discount of 10 percent off all future purchases. Now whenever Cassie needs something, she shops there first and usually finds something that will do. Her husband doesn't compliment her much anymore, and everything in her closet looks vaguely alike.

Cassie took the easy way out by confining her shopping to one place, selecting a store that specialized in "one-look dressing." Despite the discount, Cassie should shop in a larger department store or a boutique that offers more variety. There she can get to know a savvy sales associate who will help her locate the pieces she wants within the budget she has to work with, including targeting special sales to fit Cassie's level of spending. Never let habit, budget, or lack of confidence make you into a clone dresser, repeating your purchases until you become a clone even of yourself.

But wait a minute. What about Kay's bright colors and busy patterns, which she purchased to avoid the unrelieved clonedom of blacks and neutrals in her wardrobe? She wants to vary her look, yet she doesn't feel comfortable in these louder colors once she's purchased them. Or take Virginia, who had been wearing the same black pants and matching jacket once a week for two years. She needed to replace them with another suit, but she worried that black had become too blah. So she bought a red suit and a deep purple coatdress. Now Virginia notices she's still wearing the black outfit at least once every six days, and the seat of the pants and the knees are getting worn and shiny.

There's a fine line between wearing the same few things every day and purchasing styles, colors, and patterns you are uneasy wearing just because you think you should. Like Kay and Virginia, you will end up pushing these often-expensive purchases aside every time you go to your closet, reaching for that same tired ensemble while lamenting that you don't have a thing to wear! There *are* solutions to varying your wardrobe while staying true to your personal style. The women we work with learn to do just that and come away with wardrobes that make them feel attractive, comfortable, powerful, sexy, and completely themselves—every day. The strategies you'll find in chapters 3 through 5 will help you to avoid clone dressing while making the most of the real you.

CREATE A CLOTHES DIARY

What happens after you've created the Circle of Your Life and compared it to your closet? Well, it would be nice to think that changes in shopping and wearing patterns happen overnight, but in most cases this simply isn't realistic. As we have seen, the motivations for buying and wearing what we do can run deep, and it is going to take some effort to establish new and improved wardrobes in keeping with who we are. Chances are that even when you've had your closet epiphany, you'll still be tempted by impulse purchases, Someday Clothes, clone dressing, and other old habits. This is why we recommend that women follow up their Circle of Your Life with a clothes diary. After keeping this diary for three to six months and shopping for clothes within this period, you will be able to clearly see shopping patterns and needs, and can make adjustments accordingly.

Start keeping a diary of everything you buy to wear. You can keep it with you at all times by adding a notepad or index cards to your pocket calendar. If you use a notebook-style date book such as a Day-Timer or Filofax, add blank sheets in a designated Clothes Diary section in the back.

First write down the month, and then list any items purchased, the date of purchase, and their approximate cost. You want to describe each item sufficiently so you will know what it is when you look at the description six months or a year later. Bonnie, a black-belt bargain shopper, finds it helpful to write the store name beside the purchase and whether the item was regular price, on sale, or a super bargain.

After you have been keeping your diary for about six months, get three colored Magic Markers. We use pink, green, and blue. Use pink marker to highlight purchases that have become favorites—things you wear and love. Use green to highlight clothes that have now become dependables—"best friend" clothes that help form the backbone of your wardrobe. Then use blue for mistakes—things you never or rarely wear.

You will be surprised how revealing this exercise is! Many of our clients confess that their emotional purchases are costly, and that most super bargains prove instead to be super mistakes. You may also be startled to see which purchases have become your best friend basics.

Linda, a college psychologist and mother of two teenagers who lives in Chicago, must shop carefully and watch her budget. Her diary looks like this:

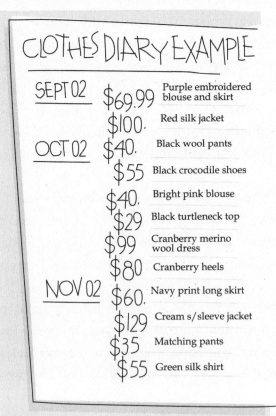

CLOTHES DIARY EXAMPLE

SEPT 02	$69.99	Purple embroidered blouse and skirt
	$100.	Red silk jacket
OCT 02	$40.	Black wool pants
	$55	Black crocodile shoes
	$40.	Bright pink blouse
	$29	Black turtleneck top
	$99	Cranberry merino wool dress
	$80	Cranberry heels
NOV 02	$60.	Navy print long skirt
	$129	Cream s/sleeve jacket
	$35	Matching pants
	$55	Green silk shirt

Throughout the three-month period that Linda kept her diary, she found herself still frustrated with her closet and her shopping. Despite keeping a record of her purchases, she still never seemed to have a thing to wear on a daily or weekly basis. Yet Linda thought she did a good job of shopping and planning ahead. Note the Christmas party purchase of a red silk jacket in September, and her November purchases in anticipation of an island vacation in January. What did Linda discover when she began analyzing her list and highlighting her favorites, dependables, and mistakes?

First, Linda was amazed to realize that her cranberry wool dress had become a real dependable, one she reached for week after week. When she originally bought the dress, she had assumed its vivid color would make it an occasional wear only. But in examining her preferences, Linda realized that the dress's simple lines, body-skimming fit, and cozy wool (for Chicago winters) made it wonderfully versatile. She immediately began shopping for a similar dress in another color or print. Linda also learned that her plan-ahead purchases were expensive and had short lives. In Chicago, a red silk jacket is not something you wear to work in winter *or* summer, so her idea of making an appropriate purchase for the holidays backfired. The resort outfit was marvelous and glamorous for her week in St. Thomas, but it was impossible to fit into her social life in Illinois. Only Linda can decide if the cost of this outfit was worth it.

YOUR PLAN

After the Circle of Your Life reveals what you are missing, make a list to help you shop right now. Then begin your clothes diary as a good follow-up to give you insight into what clothes are basics for you and what styles and colors you love to wear. Those "mistake marks" will help you realize what leads you to waste your money: often so-called bargains, impulse buys, or pushy sales clerks or friends who talk you into wearing something that is their taste.

We have added a sample clothes diary page you may photocopy or use as a format in the back of your daily appointment book. Keep your diary near your wallet, so you'll always have it handy when shopping. (We'll learn lots more about shopping strategies in chapter 9.)

Once you are well on your way, you will want to redraw the Circle of Your Life every year or two. This way you can track how your activities change, your career grows, and your personal life goes through transitions. The Circle is an immediate check on why your wardrobe isn't keeping pace with the path you have taken in your life.

The Circle of Your Life is the foundation of our plan to help you gain insight and understanding into the psychology of your closet. It's the first step toward rethinking your closet, your clothes, and your life. In the following chapters, we'll provide you with the know-how to change the way you choose and organize what you wear and, more important, the way you feel about yourself!

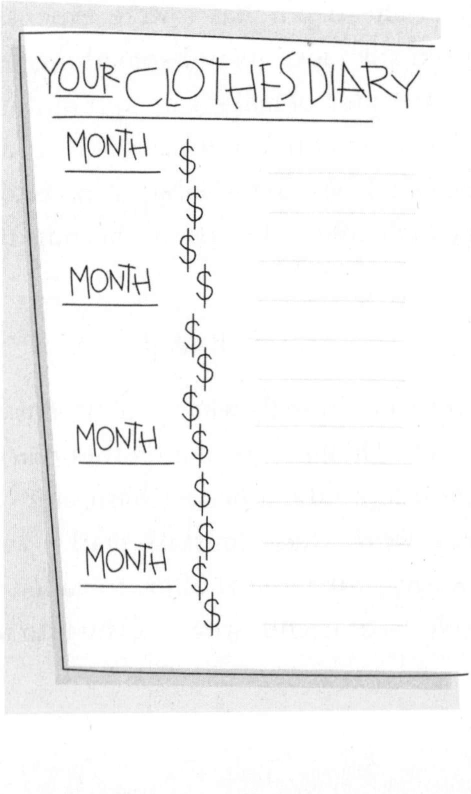

YOUR CLOTHES DIARY

MONTH $
$
$
$
MONTH $
$
$
$
MONTH $
$
$
MONTH $
$
$

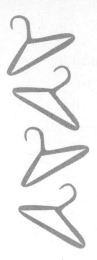

CHAPTER TWO

LET'S DEFINE YOU

Beauty is not necessarily beautiful features. It's about under-standing one's style and having the attitude to carry off that style. If a woman feels beautiful, she will make others see her as beautiful.

CHARLOTTE RAMPLING, ACTOR

Picking up this book indicates you want to know more about your-self, whether you realize it or not. This chapter will help you gain information and greater understanding about your image of your-self, your thought patterns, your inner emotions, and how your clothes and accessories play an important role in your overall self-esteem.

Let's start with a fun quiz!

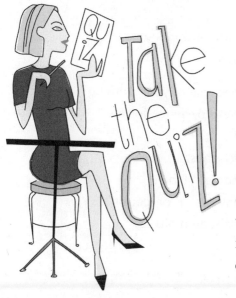

SELF-DISCOVERY QUIZ

This is designed to help you understand and define the process you use to select your clothes. It has nothing to do with your sense of personal style or your fashion personality, such as dramatic, romantic, or classic; that comes later! It is intended to provide insight on how you view yourself and the process by which you select your clothing. The clothes in your closet are a reflection of your sense of confidence and authentic self.

DIRECTIONS: Please choose the answer that reflects your most typical behavior. In other words, choose the answer that reflects what you actually do or think, NOT what you would *like* to do or feel you *should* do. All of the questions are forced choice questions. There are no right or wrong answers, and your score is based on the pattern of answers, not your answer to any particular question.

1. What best describes your feelings as a child when you shopped for clothes?
   a. I looked forward to shopping. My mother helped guide me and I liked the experience.
   b. I never went shopping. I wore whatever my mother brought home for me.
   c. I dreaded the experience and tried to avoid it.
   d. I loved it! My mom says I always had definite ideas about what I wanted to wear.

2. What best describes the way your parents, brothers or sisters, or friends described your appearance as a child?
   a. No real description. I don't remember.
   b. Beautiful, angelic, could be a model.
   c. Names such as stork, chubby, gawky, etc. A tomboy.
   d. She's going through an awkward stage.

3. Did you ever feel badly about yourself because of your clothing?
   a. No. They have always been a positive experience for me, except for one or two slipups.
   b. I don't remember. Clothes were just clothes.
   c. I always had the right clothes with the right labels.
   d. Yes, on several occasions. I wore my sister or cousin's hand-me-downs and we shopped at discount stores.

4. Was a clothing budget ever an issue for you as a child or teen?
    a. I always felt I had the minimum of what I needed to wear.
    b. I never had enough money to purchase and wear what the "in" crowd wore.
    c. No. I had lots of clothes. I was rather spoiled that way as a child.
    d. I didn't really care.

5. What do you remember about your body as a preteen between the ages of 10 to 14?
    a. I played sports and never had a weight problem.
    b. I was more interested in what I was doing and was comfortable with my body.
    c. I was chubby and used clothes as a cover-up.
    d. There were parts of my body that I considered to be a problem.

6. How do you feel about looking in mirrors?
    a. I work hard to look good and I like what I see.
    b. I check myself out once in the morning and that's it for the day.
    c. It's not my favorite thing. I constantly see my insecurities.
    d. I am constantly checking myself in every reflective surface to make sure I am okay.

7. How do you feel about having your picture taken?
    a. I don't mind. I kind of like it.
    b. I never like the way I look in pictures.
    c. If the occasion arises I do it.
    d. I avoid it at all costs, stand behind something or volunteer to take the picture.

8. When you get dressed, what factors or people do you consider?
   a. I dress to please myself. I have my own style.
   b. I dress for the situation or my career, to please my employer and represent the company to clients. On weekends, I please myself.
   c. I am confused and am constantly trying to find my appropriate personal style.
   d. I dress to please the current man in my life and men in general.

9. How do you feel your co-workers or friends judge your appearance?
   a. I follow the dress code and the rules. I like to fit in.
   b. I look successful—like a manager or executive.
   c. They always compliment me and ask my advice about clothes.
   d. I do my own creative thing.

10. Do you ever ask for advice in creating your personal wardrobe?
    a. Usually other people ask me for advice.
    b. I do my own thing.
    c. I tend to ask my husband or a friend to help narrow my decisions.
    d. Yes, frequently. I just don't know how to put it all together.

11. Have you ever had a current or past love make you feel inadequate about the way you dressed?
    a. No. If he did and it hurt my feelings, he'd be history.
    b. Occasionally. I'm sensitive.
    c. I never dated that much so it just didn't happen.
    d. At one time something like that would have bothered me, but not now.

12. In social situations do you judge your look by what others are wearing?
    a. I always call my friends to see what they are wearing before I decide.
    b. I am more interested in what I am doing than what I am wearing.
    c. I try to be understated to fit in.
    d. I change ten times before leaving the house but still don't feel I have chosen the right outfit.

13. How did you learn to put outfits together and to create a wardrobe?
    a. I am still learning. I have a personal shopper or one salesperson I really rely on.
    b. No one. Coordinating clothes has always made me feel challenged and insecure.
    c. I've always loved clothes and learned from all over: magazines, friends, relatives.
    d. Clothes or fashion were never a big priority. I just put things together that are comfortable.

14. Select one word that you feel describes your sense of dress.
    a. Confident.
    b. Adequate.
    c. Experimental.
    d. Boring.

15. Are you unhappy about the size you wear?
    a. Yes! I'm tempted to cut the size label out of my clothes as soon as I get home.
    b. I constantly fluctuate. I probably have wardrobes in several sizes in my closet.
    c. No. I work out and watch what I eat.
    d. I care about comfort and fit. Size is no issue.

16. What do you say when you receive a compliment?
    a. Thanks. I got it on sale.
    b. Thank you. It's kind of you to tell me.
    c. Do you really think so?
    d. I wish I could believe that.

17. Identify the reaction you have when one of those MTV fashion shows pops up on television, or you actually go to a fashion show.
    a. I love to watch them. I always look for tips and looks I might want to try.
    b. I feel deflated and that my fashion sense is hopeless.
    c. I have no interest in them. Those shows rarely show anything real people would want or wear.
    d. I usually like one or two outfits I can relate to.

18. How do you feel when you get on a scale?
    a. What I see usually dictates my mood for several hours.
    b. It is scary. I do make it a weekly ritual.
    c. I only get on a scale at the doctor's office.
    d. If I see a problem, I vow to do something about it, and then do it.

19. Do you shop when you go on vacation?
    a. Always. I look for special stores and clothes we don't have back home.
    b. I simply cannot drive by an outlet center without stopping and shopping for bargains.
    c. I usually pick up sports clothes such as golf or tennis gear. I like souvenir tee shirts so people will know where I've been.
    d. I look but never buy.

20. Describe how you feel when you clean out your closet.
    a. I am afraid to give things away. I buy new ones and am confused by the amount of clothing I have.
    b. I love everything and it all looks great on me. I just keep adding to it.
    c. Very objective. Unemotional. I wore it, liked it, I'm over wearing it.
    d. I give old pieces to charity, make lists, and replace with new items each season.

21. When you have to wear a swimsuit someplace, what does your inner voice say to you?
    a. All right! Now I get to show off the hard work of dieting and the hours I've spent at the gym.
    b. I'm okay with wearing a suit with friends.
    c. Good grief! I shop and shop until I find a suit that doesn't make me look too bad.
    d. I don't own a suit. I would plead a terminal illness before donning one.

22. Do you need approval from your husband or date before you feel comfortable wearing an outfit to a social event?
    a. Yes. I ask at home and then continue to ask all during the event, "Do you like this on me?"
    b. No. I trust my own taste.
    c. I may ask, but it won't affect my choice. I felt confident enough to buy shoes and jewelry to go with it.
    d. Yes. I ask and usually take the advice.

23. Do you enjoy shopping alone or would you prefer to go with friends?
    a. I am particular about who I shop with. I go mostly alone.
    b. I don't like to shop.
    c. I go with friends to make it a social event.
    d. I like to go with friends so I can solicit their opinions.

24. How do you feel about wearing a jacket?
    a. It doesn't matter. I like a jacket when it suits the style.
    b. I always wear jackets. They make me feel secure; I don't like revealing my body.
    c. I always wear a third piece: a jacket, an open cardigan, or a big shirt worn over a tee or camisole. This look is my uniform because I believe it makes my body look better than form-fitting clothes.
    d. Jackets make me feel complete, spiffy, and polished.

25. Would you say you feel good about yourself?
    a. Almost always.
    b. Never thought of it in those terms.
    c. Under construction. I have my ups and downs.
    d. I work toward this goal.

SCORING

Add up your total score based on this tally.

	a	b	c	d
1.	a-4	b-3	c-1	d-5
2.	a-3	b-5	c-1	d-2
3.	a-4	b-1	c-5	d-3
4.	a-4	b-2	c-5	d-3
5.	a-3	b-4	c-1	d-2
6.	a-4	b-5	c-1	d-2
7.	a-5	b-2	c-3	d-1
8.	a-4	b-3	c-2	d-5
9.	a-1	b-2	c-5	d-3
10.	a-5	b-3	c-2	d-1
11.	a-5	b-3	c-1	d-2

12. a-1   b-3   c-4   d-2

13. a-2   b-1   c-4   d-3

14. a-5   b-3   c-4   d-1

15. a-4   b-2   c-5   d-3

16. a-4   b-2   c-1   d-3

17. a-5   b-1   c-3   d-2

18. a-5   b-2   c-3   d-4

19. a-5   b-3   c-2   d-1

20. a-1   b-5   c-3   d-2

21. a-2   b-3   c-4   d-1

22. a-1   b-4   c-5   d-2

23. a-4   b-3   c-5   d-2

24. a-4   b-1   c-3   d-2

25. a-5   b-3   c-2   d-4

TOTAL _____

SUPERCONFIDENT—90 POINTS OR MORE

Superconfident women have a great sense of self. You are poised and believe in your abilities. Your mother and/or father built your self-esteem by creating a positive environment or by steering you to challenges that resulted in accomplishments. Your confidence could also have been hard-won, by facing up to personal difficulties or overcoming insecurities later in life. Like Barbra Streisand, if you were teased as a child about your appearance, you have overcome the faults or accepted them as uniquely yours.

Shopping for clothes is a positive experience for you. It started in your early years as you garnered compliments from family and friends.

Today, clothes represent fun and fashion. You are bold and fearless in your choices. You like to explore as you shop, and you use clothes as a means of self-expression.

A woman such as yourself, with a strong sense of style, occasionally can intimidate other women. As a superconfident woman you must be careful not to come across as conceited, cocky, or arrogant.

CONFIDENT BUT EXPERIMENTAL—75 TO 89 POINTS

You believe that one does not *find* one's self, the self is something one creates and refines by experimenting. You feel secure about your appearance and your choices. You have learned, by testing, what you like and what works for your psyche and your body. You have an image of yourself you like.

You are comfortable with the experience of shopping and putting together outfits and a workable wardrobe. You still seek out advice from time to time and scan fashion magazines occasionally to keep up with trends. You do not allow fashion to trespass on your personal boundaries, which are a part of your identity. For example: you know what length skirt is best for you, or that you would never be comfortable wearing ruffles or something "sweet."

Like education, your self-image is a life-long endeavor you intend to tweak as you move through the years. Chapter 4, Discover Your Fashion Persona—Internal Self-Expression may open your eyes to an aspect of your personality you have yet to discover.

CONTENT AND COMFORTABLE—65 TO 74 POINTS

Clothes and fashion are not all that important to you. You wear your hair short or cut in a wash-and-go style because it is easy. You like easy-care, nonconstricting clothes. Your dry cleaning bills are tiny. You wear "appropriate" things that are versatile, or you have evolved a "uniform" for yourself to eliminate stress when you dress. Coco Chanel loved the LBD (Little Black Dress), and so do you. It goes out at night whenever you do.

You see a fashion show only if the ticket proceeds benefit a charitable cause you support. You would feel dysfunctional reading fashion magazines. Shopping for clothes is prompted by need. You don't have identity issues you wish to cure through clothes and other superficial accoutrements. The French have a term, *bien dans sa peau,* which loosely translates to "comfortable in her skin."

However, you might tend to be too conservative about your appearance and actually be missing some of the fun that can be found in fashion. Beware of letting your look become anonymous or boring. Check out chapter 4, Discover Your Fashion Persona— Internal Self-Expression, and also chapter 6 on body proportions. Women often discover from these two discussions that evaluations made long ago about themselves or their bodies are incorrect or outdated. Looking at yourself with "fresh eyes" could open up exciting possibilities for you.

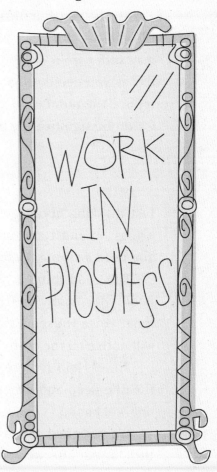

WORK IN PROGRESS—50 TO 64 POINTS

Image issues plague memories of your early years. You ate too many cookies and didn't make cheerleader. Your mother insisted you have a perm every six months. You were five feet eleven inches tall at age eleven. Your family struggled financially and your hand-me-down clothes sucked. You were smart and a nerd. All this makes you determined to be your finest and best today.

You study well-dressed, successful women to learn their secrets; you pore over fashion magazines; you try a new hairstyle every few months; and you are a cosmetic junkie. You know in detail how every "hot" diet works. You've been color analyzed and "made over." You love to have your makeup done at cosmetic counters at the beginning of each season. You may have hired a personal shopper to help you enhance or define who you are.

The danger lies in obsession. Change is not always an improvement. Be aware when you hit the right thing for *you,* such as your perfect hairstyle, and stick with it. Moderate ongoing attention to self-improvement is a good thing.

As this quiz indicates some indecision on your part, chapter 5, Closetology 101, can assist with editing your current wardrobe, which may suffer from an abundance of choices you must wade through each day as you decide what to wear. Chapter 11 on traveling could help you reduce the number of suitcases you take along by helping you edit your wardrobe significantly before your next trip.

HELP!—49 POINTS OR FEWER

Just thinking about getting dressed for a major event or job interview brings on angst and anxiety attacks. Your diagnosis: confidence issues. You need a strong prescription to prop up your self-esteem.

The good thing is, you know you need help. Way back in your childhood your family or friends beat up on your ego, and ever since, your inner voice whispers urgently, "Keep your head down, hide, and no one will notice all the stuff that is wrong with you."

Piffle! Help is here in the pages of this book. We are here for you. Breathe deep and dive in. If you reread a chapter two or three times, no one will know.

We designed this as a long-term reference book—a source you can turn to year after year, whenever you need a wardrobe "tune-up."

SELF-KNOWLEDGE IS THE KEY

The knowledge you've just uncovered about yourself is relevant to you here and now. Throughout your life you evolve and change, and this is both a challenge and a privilege. The privilege is our priceless opportunity to grow in knowledge and experience. Challenges occur through maturation, self-motivation, advancement, and catastrophe.

Personal calamities are powerful instigators forcing change and growth, such as what happened to Lorna, a consultant in Southern California. Self-knowledge is sometimes hard earned.

"About three years ago I was living with the man of my dreams," she said. *"After we started going together, I quit my job, helped him entertain clients, went to lunch with girl-*

"Self-knowledge is key to dressing from the inside out."

friends, and went shopping. Oh, I did lots of shopping. I was on the lounge chair of life. Then one afternoon he came home and said, 'We have to talk.' And my world collapsed. Soon he married another woman."

After several months, Lorna sought help from a counselor and spent her early sessions wallowing in self-pity. Soon the counselor/life coach confronted her with reality: "Do you want people to see you as a pitiful person? Is that how you want to be perceived?" She assured him that was not her self-image, but she said, "I don't know what I should do." He said, "You need to lose weight, get your professional appearance back, and get a job, or in a few years you are going to find yourself an overweight, unhappy woman living alone on welfare." Lorna raged, burst into tears, and stormed out of his office. After driving a few miles she stopped at a Shop 'n Go to get a soft drink. Standing in line, she noticed the cashier's tee shirt, which read, "The truth shall set you free but first it's going to really p—— you off." That was Lorna's moment of self-realization.

She went home, created a business plan, enrolled in a diet program, and now has her own consulting business.

Her life coach gave her a prescription for a life "makeover." Most women seek to create such change on their own, either because they can't afford professional advice or because they are personally motivated. When women seek out "makeovers" from a professional, whether a complete cosmetic change in their face and hair, or a wardrobe analysis from us, we always ask, "Why? What prompted you to do this?"

Women may simply desire a new look. Curiosity or impulse is common. Deeper motivations vary, from a vague restlessness, to boredom, to emotional turmoil created by a new job, an engagement, a move to a new city, or involvement in a new relationship. Passages from one life role to another or to a different environment provoke swirls of emotions. Big changes that take a long time, such as a weight change or earning a degree, are emotionally significant.

Ambitious women may suddenly find themselves in the public or business spotlight, urged by circumstance to look professional and pulled together. Women under stress come for wardrobe and closet makeovers because they are overwhelmed and unable to deal with a jumbled mess alone.

Or you may want a makeover because it is fun and you want to satisfy your curiosity; you're an information gatherer with a love of learning new things (especially about yourself) and new ways of putting things together. Then there are women frozen in "stall" mode—people like Sara, a district attorney, who said, "Jackie, you've got to come help me gut my closet. I can't give myself permission to get rid of anything."

TRANSITIONS AND PERSONAL GROWTH

Take time for self-discovery. See if you recognize any of the motivations below as being a factor in your life, and add others that could be making a difference in your emotions right now.

- You've moved to a new city or neighborhood
- You found a wonderful new job or got promoted
- You just met an intriguing new man
- Your husband was promoted
- A body change—weight gain or loss
- Illness
- Relationship changes—divorce, breakup, a readjustment
- Stress
- Being bored or having the desire for a change—wanting a "makeover"
- Feeling overwhelmed; the process seems too complicated to tackle
- _____
- _____
- _____

We are all ongoing works in progress. This interactive chapter uses soul-searching as a means to help you learn truths about yourself and perhaps confront personal issues that may be holding you back from realizing, understanding, and committing to becoming all that you want to be. Our aim is to help you see yourself differently—not as you were yesterday, but as who you are today.

You may be surprised to learn that the image you have of yourself might not be what the world sees.

Maeve Binchy, author of Circle of Friends *and other books, tells of being at a wedding reception and seeing a woman through a glass door. "I saw a pleasant, smiling, plump, middle-aged woman coming toward me. She wore a coat and dress and a ridiculous hat. . . . I moved to open the door for her, but then I discovered there was no door. I had been looking in a mirror." Her first reaction was amazement, then realization. "I had thought I looked totally different."*

Cosmetic surgeons say women often come to them for face-lifts or other procedures after catching unexpected glimpses of themselves in store windows, snapshots, or mirrors. This disconcerting reality, different from what they see at home while positioned in a familiar way before a mirror, startles them. We are not suggesting surgery, but rather a change in perception of who you actually are today. Occasionally you need to take a fresh look at you.

ESTEEM ISSUES— GETTING TO THE HEART OF THE MATTER

Every day different stories are created in our lives, and we tend to use clothing to enhance, solve, or salve these emotional situations. Your feelings about your wardrobe are emotional. When you bought each item, you made a conscious selection. Clothes are inanimate objects. They didn't leap off the rack pleading a case as to why you should adopt them and give them a home. Like a courtship, your first experiences with a piece of clothing may be exciting. The relationship continues smoothly, then one day you realize the thrill is gone. You need a change, something new in your life.

Reasons for your disenchantment may be based in your feelings of self-esteem. You rely on your clothes as emotional props. If you feel a dress you loved isn't flattering anymore, it could be those extra pounds you've gained, a vague depression brought on by a totally unrelated experience, or a change in how much you like a particular season or certain weather. But most women we know blame their clothes. It's easier to think something happened to the dress, or, "I never noticed this blouse did that before." And the solution is always, "Let's go to the mall." When women find no comfort in their closet they go shopping and continue making the same mistakes, or they come home frustrated after buying nothing.

The answer to your dilemma is inside you.

Robin, a community activist in Nebraska, expounded her theory one fall: "Have you noticed how your sweaters seem to shrink in storage?" Or perhaps, you had an experience like Betty's: "After I turned forty-six, I woke up one morning and found that someone had taken my body in the middle of the night. My daughter has my body, and I was left with one that droops in all the wrong places." The sad truth is, nothing in your closet fits the body you suddenly found yourself living in.

> "You rely on your clothes as emotional props."

Perceived figure problems have sneaky ways of suddenly appearing when you least expect them. Last year a skirt looked great, this year there's something weird about it. Why are the buttons on your favorite white shirt suddenly gaping and straining?

Last spring, Mindy was captivated by a pantsuit in a lovely shade of pink. The color called out to her in the store. She charged it, took it home, and wore it that very night. Two days later she wore it again. The third time, she twirled in front of her full-length mirror and stopped dead. "WHAT was I thinking? From the back, I look like a big block of Bazooka bubble gum."

Do any of these incidents sound familiar? It gets worse. You know you need to get rid of the item. But then separation anxiety rears its ugly head, whipping you with thoughts like, "That dress (coat, jacket, sweater) cost a lot of money, money you are going to throw away." "You can't give that away to charity. Your sister (mother, husband) gave it to you as a gift." "I don't care if you wore it the day you got divorced (fired, heart broken, betrayed). It's still perfectly good. Just get over it."

Your closet is full of memories of good times in your life and bad. Why keep reminders of bad events in front of you each morning?

Be strong. Get rid of that stuff. You'll feel better.

AGE ISN'T WHAT IT USED TO BE

Judie wrote a profile about Dorrie, a forty-something counseling psychologist at a university, and ran into a problem. "My editor at the time was a bear about including people's ages in all such stories, and Dorrie refused to tell me how old she was." Dorrie's explanation was simple. "I don't tell people how old I am because people immediately make assumptions about you and your life that are age related and usually not very flattering."

Every day, the issue of age is in your face. Charges of "age bias" fly at Hollywood executives for failing to cast female actors in films after they reach thirty-five. Fashion and cosmetic companies blithely talk about models with "expired use-by" ages, signaling their over-the-hill status. Cosmetic ads pitch age-defying or "lift" products next to magazine stories highlighting the best cosmetic surgeons in America.

How you feel about your age and its implications have an important impact on how you feel about yourself and ultimately how you look, dress, and present yourself to the world.

For decades women believed in life stages and traditional fashion rules, such as designer-dictated hemlines, no sleeveless dresses after thirty-seven, and not wearing white shoes after Labor Day. Some women still believe them. Are you one of them?

Women's magazines used to line up neatly according to a reader's *age and life stage.* At about eleven or twelve as a preteen, you read *YM* (Young Miss), *Jane,* or *Seventeen.* As a teenager, your attention shifted to *Mademoiselle* and *Glamour.* In the late teens or your early twenties, *Cosmo* and *In Style* made inroads. Later you start picking up *Ladies' Home Journal, Redbook,* or *Marie Claire.* Then if your sophistication and worldliness expanded, your attention shifted to *Vogue* and *Harper's Bazaar.*

Not anymore! Assumptions about age and traditional life stages are disappearing. A woman of forty-five today could be a new bride, the mother of teenagers, a grandmother, or off to Tuscany on vacation with a live-in lover.

The physical fitness revolution launched in the 1980s and continuing today produces legions of women whose bodies and appearance defy their calendar age. *Lisa K, a client devoted to workouts and participating in 10K and marathon runs, is typical. During a shopping trip, the forty-seven-year-old told Jackie she had the taste level of a thirty-year-old because she knew she could wear body-conscious clothes. "I don't, of course, because of peer pressure about how a woman of my age should dress. Yet it is almost impossible to find things I like and want to wear. I work hard to look like this."*

"Today it's attitude, not age."

ATTITUDE, INTERESTS, AND PSYCHOGRAPHICS

Women's interests today transcend age boundaries. And women of any age feel overwhelmed at having too much to do and too little time to do it. You can be stressed at twenty-two, thirty-seven, or fifty-four. Stress is a *psychographics feature* transcending age or gender. Women of any age are also interested in inner spirituality, shopping, dating, home decor, sex, physical fitness, or active sports. Each interest, in the eyes of marketers, is a *psychographic* defining a group with a shared interest or concern.

In 2001, demographic researchers released a study on women's relationships to media and magazines. In the turbulent economic environment of the dot-com stock market meltdown, women's magazines emerged as the most effective media for reaching female consumers. The reason? Women's magazines, more than television, the Internet, or any other media, kept up with the trends changing women's lives.

More remarkable was the demise of magazines for women based on age clusters, such as *Mademoiselle.* At the same time those magazines failed, new ones emerged that focused on lifestyle and psychographics. Today a woman is attracted to magazines that appeal to her emotionally and reflect her lifestyle. *Attitude prevails, not an age.* That's why a single forty-seven-year-old will pick up *Cosmopolitan,* while a twenty-five-year-old with two small children chooses *Good Housekeeping* or *Better Homes and Gardens.*

Yes, sex and fashion are still in your face at the checkout line, but so are *O, The Oprah Magazine; More;* and *Real Simple* magazine. *O,* with a circulation of two million, took off like a rocket, finding appeal with women of all ages in its mix of spiritual calm, self-help pop psychology, and lively features highlighted by a monthly Oprah interview with a timely newsmaker or celebrity. *Real Simple,* Zen-like in layout, struck a chord with readers from ages twenty-six to fifty-four with its timeless advice, short-cut cookery, and timesaving housekeeping, plus an emphasis on simple organization skills.

More magazine, another success story, grew out of a need to address baby boomer women. It appeals to the mature woman who feels young, looks young, and is young in attitude. Even AARP (American Association for Retired People) split their *Modern Maturity* magazine into two parts, with one appealing to senior mature people and the second, *My Generation,* appealing to younger mature readers. Even more interesting, AARP adopted a new motto, "Live your life, not your age."

Today's sixty-year-old was only forty when MTV exploded. Fifty-something mothers often sit down with their twenty-year-old offspring and watch the same videos or television programs—including *Sex and the City.* Stow the rocking chairs. Old people aren't your little granny and grandpop anymore. Old-fogey-dom is gone.

Is your thinking tuned in to this change?

Women frequently tell us strikingly similar stories. They are walking through a mall or down a street of shops, and an outfit catches their eye. They stop, admire it, then hear a tiny voice in their brain: "You can't wear that. Your friends would think you've lost your mind," or "You're too old to wear that. Women your age shouldn't dress in styles like that." These are echoes of that old way of thinking. But a new era is here.

FINANCES AND THE SIZE OF YOUR CLOSET

The fiercest bogeyman hiding in your closet could be money. Not the lack of money or spending too much, but your relationship with money. As you grow up, emotional feelings about money create anxieties, feelings of unworthiness and fear. Are these spooks from the past still affecting you? We see manifestations of past financial experiences in women's closets all too frequently.

We firmly believe dressing well does not depend on large wardrobe allowances. Money does not magically make you well dressed. At lavish and expensive charity balls and the Academy Awards, you always see women in ghastly outfits. It's so universal that even popular magazines make sport with features about "best and worst dressed" and pictures showing hapless "fashion victims."

It doesn't take a lot of money to dress well; it just takes the right pieces. Once you learn the art of putting the pieces together, basics can be found at all price levels. Thousands of women with "black belts" in bargain shopping look marvelous. Hey, it's chic to brag about how little you spent on new clothes! Even beauteous Blaine Trump of *that* Trump family exults about casual clothes she bought the first time she visited a Target store.

But some women (you, perhaps) just don't buy that. If they don't have money to spend on beautiful clothes, their self-esteem suffers. It's the "I am not worthy" syndrome.

Karen, twenty-six, graduated from law school, landed a job with a prestigious law firm, and moved to Chicago. "The downside was my salary. It was not great. I just knew I was not measuring up to what I thought were designer-dressed associates, and every day, I started off with feel-

ings of inferiority and dread. I placed self-imposed barriers between me, my career, and business relationships."

Geraldine, a young corporate wife, echoes those feelings of inadequacy: "When we are invited to events at the grand old establishment country club or one of those stuffy, old-line private clubs, I panic. I just know all the other women there are turned out in Prada, Oscar, or Herrera dresses."

Both Karen and Geraldine are listening to their own negative-speak. This self-generated put-down demeans you. It is based on false assumptions that erect imaginary nonverbal barriers between you and other people.

One day Karen went shopping with two other women lawyers in her firm. She was surprised to learn they also operate on tight budgets, and their polished looks were purchased on sale or in discount stores.

The first management convention Geraldine and her husband attended, she learned a valuable truth about other corporate wives—a favorite outing for them during these conferences is a day spent shopping at a huge nearby discount mall. *"All those women are affluent, yet here they are fighting over half-price dresses and struggling to carry all their booty back to the hotel,"* she said.

It is true that fabric, construction, and a designer name on a label elevate the price of clothing. Yet due to the magic of "knockoffs," or copies, the look shows up and can be purchased at almost any price level. Watch the store displays just after the Academy Awards. You'll see copies of film star's gowns, priced at just several hundred dollars, appearing within days of the event.

Money spent on clothing is relative. One woman may spend $1,500 for a jacket and feel that's okay. Another may spend $100 and feel that is extravagant. Though the decision is influenced by the size of each woman's bank balance, it is still an emotional decision. Some women need the comfort or confidence a designer label gives them, while other women would only spend *x* amount of money on an item regardless of income. It is a deeply personal choice based on your history and the relationship you've had with clothing for your entire life.

Self-esteem is not linked to wardrobe size. We have seen hundreds of closets, from tiny, dark ones in two-hundred-year-old homes to room-size versions with moving, dry cleaner–type racks. We know women with only fifty-five or sixty pieces hanging in their closets, but they love each and every piece and can create hundreds of outfits with them. Yet more often we see enormous walk-in closets the size of studio apartments filled with masses of clothing—and the woman living there can't get it together and says, **"I don't have a thing to wear!"**

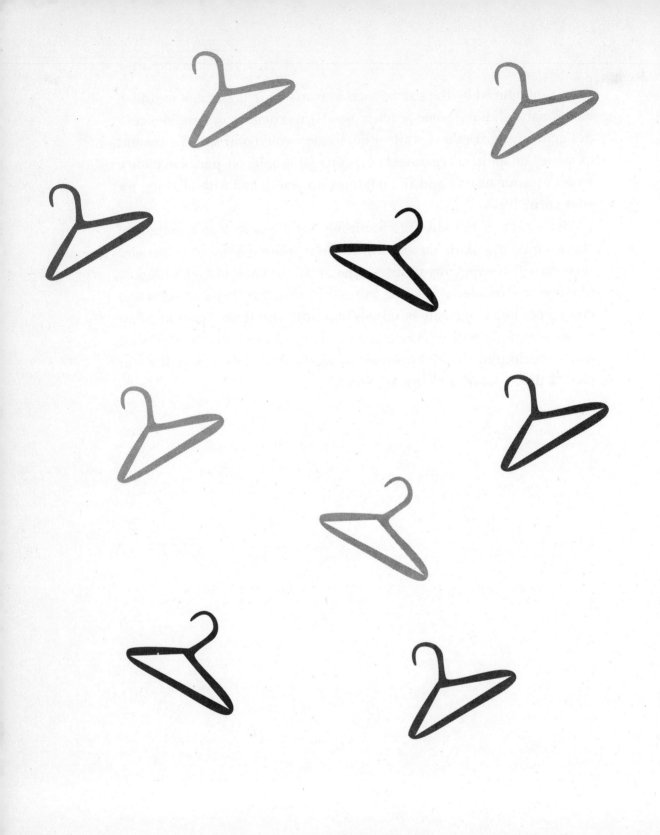

CHAPTER THREE

THE PSYCHOLOGY OF YOUR CLOSET

Eventually I managed to cheer Mum up by allowing her to go through my wardrobe and criticize all my clothes, then tell me why I should start getting everything from Jaeger and Country Casuals.

HELEN FIELDING
BRIDGET JONES'S DIARY

E ach morning you get up, brush your teeth, have your coffee, and go to your closet looking for something to wear. We go into that closet seeking what will make us *feel* our best for whatever is on the day's agenda.

As you scan your clothes, you ask, "How do I want the world to see me today?" As you make selections *you are seeking clothes that will make you feel good about yourself, and give you confidence.* It's simple. If you look as good as you can, you will feel better and *be better* out in the world.

You are not looking for an outfit; you are looking for a dose of self-esteem.

It happens each time you approach your closet, regardless of where you live, what you do, where you are going, and even if you are the only person you are going to see.

How many mornings have you tried on one outfit after another, trying to find one that "feels" right? You keep trying, and then stop in frustration. "There's nothing in here!"

One day you want to look authoritative, yet approachable. Another day you want to feel sharp, in command, up-to-the-minute; you may be

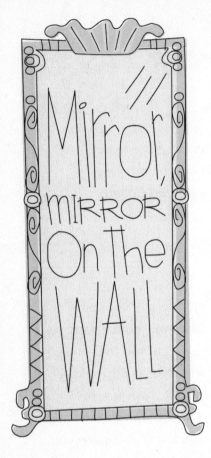

challenged by an agenda with an important business lunch or dinner with company executives. Monday you feel a need to dress "slim" to assuage your conscience for a weekend of overindulgence. Thursday evening, you may want to look sexy and attractive. Saturdays you want to coddle yourself.

The closet is a room of emotion.

Your closet houses a collective of your likes and dislikes, your past lives. Closets reveal marriages, divorces, romantic encounters, sexual attitudes, economic conditions, weight losses and gains, job changes, career paths, and even personality adjustments.

Anyone who peeks into your closet can discover your favorite colors, choices of sports, your approximate age, special interests, the sophistication of your social life, and how you spend your days.

A DAILY SEARCH FOR SELF-ESTEEM

What you select to wear projects who you are—your aspirations and your image of yourself. That can be scary, frustrating, or a boost to your self-confidence.

The clothes in your closet become costumes you assemble to play the role you want to play each day or night of your life. And those clothes reveal a great deal about how you see yourself and about things happening in your life.

Before business executives and community activists head out to an important meeting, they rely on their newest or most expensive suits to give them a look or feel of assurance. Others reach for dependable standbys or "lucky suits" because they fit well, look professional, and allow them to focus on their agenda rather than on their physical appearance. Each type of clothing provides the assurance they need to function at a top level.

Feeling better sometimes means being comforted by the familiar snuggle of a favorite sweater, or being caressed by fabrics such as jersey, silk, lamb's wool, or cashmere. On lazy days and weekends at home, when you pull on your softest sweatshirt and knit pants, you are seeking comfort and contentment.

We use clothes to help overcome insecurities about our appearance and our abilities. And we use clothes to help us "fit in" and feel more confident in certain social situations.

"You are not looking for an outfit; you are looking for a dose of self-esteem."

Whole categories of dress are shorthand designations for a look identifying a mode of dress that defines members of a group: ladies who lunch, rock stars, corporate wives, bikers, country club golfers, country singers, Palm Beach types, surfers, soccer moms. Each designation immediately conjures up a mental image of how that type of individual dresses. High school and college campuses are notorious for sartorial prejudices. Some campuses are hip-hop, some preppy; many are awash in status logos. Any new student instantly senses the vibes when their clothes are wrong.

Emulating the way other people dress in a preferred group makes *you* feel more comfortable, accepted, and perhaps hip, chic, sophisticated, or at ease.

SECRETS AND REVELATIONS

For a fun experiment, ask friends, "What would your closet reveal about your life and you?" You'll get some truly funny answers!

Most people respond with dismay at the idea of *anyone* looking in their closet. Some secretly consider it the scariest room in their house. If the question puzzles them, probe with, "Do you have a collection of tee shirts or polo shirts? What do they say on them or what is printed on them?" Chances are those shirts are embellished with travel destinations, golf resort logos, or symbols of favorite sports or rock stars. You can get into some lively conversations with your friends once they realize that items in their closet are keys to their personality quirks.

Pant style pegs a woman's place on the great age divide. Young girls live in jeans. Hip huggers hang in the closet of teen girls or a twenty-something club kid. Pull-on pants with elastic waists broadcast birth dates in another decade. And there's the flat front or pleated pants issue.

Another personality tip-off is color. Color is emotional. Favorite colors make you smile; colors you hate make you grimace just pronouncing their names. You gravitate toward wearing favorite colors on days when you feel great or have fun destinations. You decorate your house or apartment in colors appealing to you. Your *right* colors lift your spirits, set off your eyes, and make you feel more attractive.

Here's a simple color experiment that can be quite revealing, particularly for New York women, many of whom live in black clothes. In your closet, take everything black and hang it together in one spot by classification—dresses, pants, tops, skirts, etc. Is anything left in your closet? Often, people who wear black constantly are trying to hide something or "disappear." Many excuse this predilection by insisting that black is the chicest choice—but it is also the safest. After removing all black items, examine what remains, noting the preponderance of particular colors as tip-offs to your color personality.

> I think I'm going to have to stop wearing all black. . . . That's all they wear at these trendy hotels. I don't want someone to confuse me for a bellhop.
>
> KARL LAGERFELD, FASHION DESIGNER

TRUTHFULLY—WHAT PERCENTAGE OF YOUR CLOTHES DO YOU WEAR?

Now, a big question: what percentage of your clothes do you actually wear? 20 percent? 50 percent? 75 percent? Women in our seminars mostly answer 20 percent.

Men wear 90 percent of the clothes in their closets. That's because men shop by need. Women hit the stores for a variety of reasons: entertainment, boredom, to feel better, as part of an outing with friends, or to get together with sisters or your mom.

Watch a man shop. He buys six pairs of socks, a dozen boxer shorts, four dress shirts, three polo shirts, two suits, three casual pants, and perhaps four ties. He shops two, three, or only four times a year for himself.

Most women shop at the drop of a charge card.

What motivates her? Before a vacation or when everything is in the laundry, she buys panties or thongs. When she is shopping for a birthday gift for her friend, she also buys herself a blouse. On a lunch hour, she scoops up three things on sale because they are such great buys. Is it any wonder women only wear 20 percent of what's in their closet?

THE MIRROR AND INSECURITIES

We stress the importance of everyone taking one last look in a full-length mirror each time they dress to go out into the world. It is a positive step—a way of assuring that everything looks great and nothing is amiss—front, back, and sideways. When you dress in clothes that make you feel good and reflect your personality, your competence, and your life, it shows.

Too often women look in the mirror and see distortions—insecurities reflected back. Their gaze automatically goes straight to defects, real and imagined—figure flaws, facial blemishes, unruly hair, things that poke out, and things that are too flat. A few women say looking in the mirror is so painful they avoid it. Some only look in their medicine cabinet mirrors.

Women look at themselves in the mirror, and see every flaw.
Men look and see perfection.

ART COOPER, EDITOR IN CHIEF, *GQ* MAGAZINE

Social attitudes conspire to make how you look exceptionally important. Society values us as women one minute and devalues us the next.
Looking beautiful, looking better, looking younger, is an inescapable
theme song throughout a woman's life. Women are subjected to intense
media hype and shown daily doses of how to lose weight or have the right
hairstyle, how to attract or keep a man, how to wear makeup and be the
best we can be.

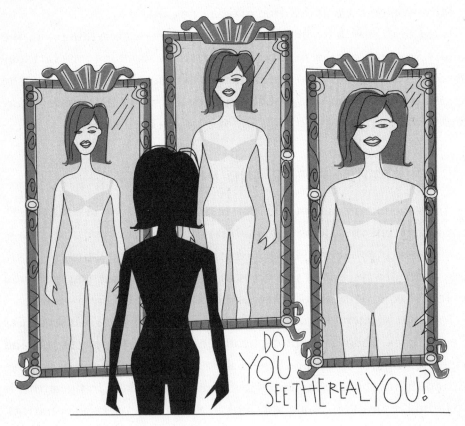

As a consequence, issues about size have reached epidemic proportions. Women feel insecure about the size, shape, and weight of their bodies. Each day, bone-thin television personalities electronically drop into our homes. Movie actresses vie to be a size 2. Oscar nominee Renée Zellweger confides in a *Vogue* magazine interview that a big dinner for her consists of "egg whites and spinach salad." Yet a figure chart in 2001 reveals the average American woman is a size 14.

In grocery checkout lines, women come face-to-face with *Us* or *People* magazine's periodic cover stories on the "current" (skinny) look of celebrity body shapes.

In our workshops, 10 percent of the women say they cut the size tags out of their clothes to avoid having to deal with that information on a daily basis.

In his *Body Image Workbook,* T. F. Cash presents a table documenting three U.S. surveys on body image conducted in 1972, 1985, and 1996. These reveal that overall body size dissatisfaction increased from 23 percent to 56 percent for women, and from 15 percent to 43 percent for men from 1972 to 1996.

"The percentages most certainly have increased even further," says Kevin Thompson, Ph.D., a psychologist and author of two books. In his work at the University of

"The closet is a room of emotion."

South Florida he specializes in body image disturbances. "There are compelling cultural forces at work distorting realistic appearances and people's perception of their own image. The media's repetitive presentation of size 2 celebrities and the new muscular trend among male models and actors in magazines such as *GQ, Details,* and *Esquire* is perpetuating an unrealistic ideal body image."

Mike, a male model in a famous designer underwear advertisement, said he would never do it again. "It was too hard. I had to eat a special diet for two months to get my body fat down to about 8 percent, plus work out six hours a day," he said. "Man, it wasn't worth it."

In addition, photographers and editors use computers to touch up final photographs and employ sophisticated lighting to further create illusions of perfection. Mike's mom, Briana, said when the ad came out, "I didn't even recognize my own son."

The cosmetic, personal care, and fashion magazine industries are built on a base of identifying women's defects. Of course, the cosmetic/beauty/fashion people have products and services designed to fix or cure these imperfections. Flip through any women's magazine and glance at the advertisements. Advertising copywriters have invented an improbable array of flaws and problems that—surprise!—can only be solved by their client's product.

In a review of the 2002 film *Legally Blonde,* critic David Denby writes in *The New Yorker* about a women's magazine: "The July issue offers confidence-building tips ('Feel Sexier Naked—Now'), but on a nearby page there are more anxieties than can be found in all of *Fear and Trembling.* Health crises loom everywhere: cold sores, bikini line breakouts. Terrifying questions are posed: 'Are your breasts unbalanced?' 'Is it bad to wash my face during a hot shower?' The magazine seems eager to trap women in a perpetual limbo of desire and fear."

Other confidence destroyers for women are those annual swimsuit issues, followed by charts in women's magazines advising "swimsuits for every figure." These present the best swimsuit choices for women with large busts, small busts, ample hips, short legs, short torso, long torso, thick torso, tummy bulge, and full (as opposed to ample) hips. This is not exactly a complimentary lineup of body shapes.

All these negative connotations and images swirl in a woman's subconscious, distorting the lens through which she sees herself.

HOW YOUR PAST POISONED
YOUR WELL OF CONFIDENCE

Like a haunted house, your closet may house a veritable flock of ghosts from your distant past. In twenty years of working in fashion and image workshops, we have met countless women who tell us they cannot wear a particular color or a style or even item of jewelry because "my mother always told me I couldn't wear green (or gold or navy or pink)" or "my mother told me that style wasn't good for my body" or "my mother told me never to wear rings or a bracelet, because my fingers and hands are too chubby." Often these women are thirty-five, forty, or even fifty years old.

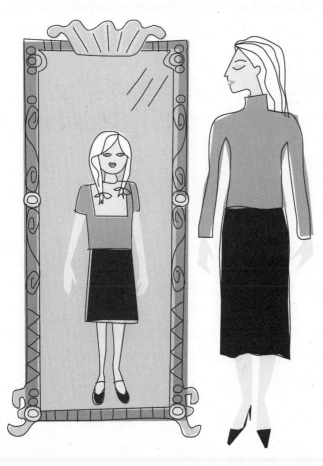

Their perception of themselves is still governed by things their mother told them when they were five, eight, twelve, or fifteen years old.

At an early age, girls learn from mothers, siblings, or friends that certain of their body's parts are flawed and imperfect, thus they must be hidden, deemphasized, or treated as major problems. Large busts are hidden under high necklines and loose-fitting blouses or shirts. Less-than-shapely legs must be covered with pants or long skirts. Hips and thunder thighs vanish beneath baggy skirts or jeans. And years later, decades later, after bodies have developed and changed, those whispers still echo in their heads. These young women, now grown, are self-conscious about figure flaws that may no longer exist.

Recently a client came to Jackie with a rather unusual request. "I want you to help me look sexy. I've never felt I dress that way."

Jackie went to Jill's closet, and there were no skirts, just pants and pantsuits. "Why is this?" Jackie asked.

"My legs are ugly. My mother told me I always had to cover them up by wearing pants, so I've worn pants all my life," said Jill.

Common sense tells you that wearing pants all your life is not a way to look sexy, but that was not the issue. We've learned most women wear pantsuits to "cover" their bodies from neck to ankle. This poor woman was forty-three years old and had never—not once in her life—felt sexy.

Jackie counseled her to wear a sexy open shoe such as a high-heeled sandal, and a low-cut tank or halter-style top or bustier, either under her jacket or without the jacket. Presto! Jill looked and felt sexy.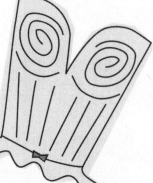

Mothers and fathers often, without thinking, script their children's future concerns by saying things obliquely: "with your height," "you're too lanky to wear——," "Jana is too chubby to wear a cheerleader skirt," "poor Karen is built just like her aunt Patricia," or "Darling, you are just not built to——." Height and weight are monitored literally from birth.

Parents fill children's lives with "should" and "shouldn't" statements that seem trivial at the time yet echo decades later in a woman's vision of herself. Your past reaches into your present.

My mom was a model and an actress, and she knew what was beautiful. She would say, "Your eyes are too close together, so when you put your eyeliner on you have to draw the lines up here, like this, because your eyes are already too small and your face is too wide, and see, honey, you have your father's mouth. I don't know if I would have known how beautiful she was, if she wasn't always pointing out how unbeautiful I was.

JENNIFER ANNISTON, ACTOR

Sometimes a mother's criticism isn't intended as such, but girls hear a different message in their hearts.

Kristen, thirty-eight, told us her mother would say things like, "Kristen, you should find out where Kathy buys her clothes. She always looks so nice." Or her mother picked up Seventeen *and showed Kristen pictures of hairstyles or clothes with the recommendation "You should try these, dear. They are very in for young people."*

"I always felt like she was telling me my clothes looked awful, and implying that Kathy knows how to dress and I don't," said Kristin. "She was always critical about the way I looked."

Mothers may be trying to be helpful. But these comments are not heard that way.

Your mom may have worked so hard to dress you well, make your hair look good, and have you achieve great things, because she wanted her friends to think she was a good parent. *It had nothing to do with your shortcomings.*

Often these parental remarks come during the early teens, a time when young people are seeking their identities, experimenting with their looks, and plagued with self-doubt. Their parents' apparent disapproval only feeds a young person's insecurities.

In childhood and beyond, peers and friends point out your big ears or pointed nose, small chin, haystack hair, extended height, puny build, geeky glasses, clumsy walk, fat body, skinny body, bow legs, big feet, flat chest, or protruding elbows. Then they dream up nicknames for you. These cruel and thoughtless taunts remain deep in our hearts and emerge as shadows of insecurity each time we look in the mirror at our image. These events create fixed beliefs about your appearance.

Jackie remembers her father taking her on a shopping trip when she was eleven. "We were on a strict family budget, but he took me to a famous-name department store in Philadelphia. We picked out two 'dream come true' outfits for me. The next day I proudly wore one to school, a red and cream striped sweater with a red skirt. While changing classes, one of the most popular guys in school looked at me and said, 'Hey, chubby! Boy, are those big stripes.' I went home and hid that sweater so far back in my closet I didn't find it for years. Today it is still hard for me to buy stripes."

Everyone was jeered at, teased, and mocked about something when they were a child, whether from friends or family members, but few realize this is a universal situation. Instead women coddle their hurts as unique to them alone, and for years they see themselves as inadequate and imperfect. This condition is a psychic disfigurement, a failing to understand that unfortunate things people said to you way back in the fifth grade are distorting the way you see yourself today.

Begin to listen to what you are telling yourself. Ask, "Where did that idea come from?" If you trace it to your childhood, get rid of it. You are stuck in a perception of yourself based in history, an impression other people have given you about who you are.

FLASHBACKS CAN SET YOU FREE

Looking back to your past and remembering difficult situations may help you gain understanding about negative attitudes you have about yourself.

One way to help is by looking at old pictures. Like many people, you may laugh at how you used to look or be profoundly embarrassed. Celebrities and movie actors must cringe when they see their high school pictures in current magazines; almost anyone would. Realizing that a great statesman once looked like a geek or that beauties once had buckteeth, ghastly hairdos, and chubby bodies should help you realize that everyone's appearance grows and changes. Understanding this fact can be a gift of revelation and insight. *Your history is not your destiny.*

For a different flashback, think about where you lived. Geographical roots often manifest themselves in clothes and personal preferences. Can you imagine Dolly Parton without her country music hairdo and clothes? Could George W. Bush or Robert Redford be comfortable without their western boots?

People who love the great outdoors dress differently than urbanites do. Coastal dwellers and sailors savor nautical traditions and functional looks associated with life on deck, by beaches, harbors, and bays.

Places you live even for a short period of time can influence your tastes for years to come. What are your roots and former addresses, and how do they influence you today?

Your family's economic condition in your childhood also often casts long shadows over your style and attitudes today.

Rosemary, a prominent attorney and a self-made mover and shaker in state politics, confesses she crams the closets of each of her four homes (urban, beach, condo in the state capital, and ski chalet) with clothes. "I have huge closets, and they are all stuffed," she said. "I grew up in a family with very little money and all my clothes came from the Salvation Army thrift store. I've never gotten over it."

A more common symptom of growing up with limited means is an inability to throw anything away. Clothes age in closets because a woman recalls how much they cost and cannot "throw away" or part with the item.

A woman reared in plush circumstances may exhibit a preference for fine fabrics and designer clothes. At the end of each season, her clothes are promptly whisked off to a consignment store.

Which media stars did you admire growing up? Did you try to copy their hairstyle, like the millions of girls who tortured their tresses into Farrah Fawcett flips in the 1980s or a *Friends* shag in the 1990s?

Did you get your fashion cues from Gwyneth Paltrow, Julia Roberts, Diane Keaton, Doris Day, Audrey Hepburn, or Grace Kelly? Did you copy their clothes or emulate their style? Characters in movies occasionally prompt imitation.

Or MTV may have been an influence, causing you to pierce your ears five times, wear ripped jeans, or bare your midriff.

> The clothes you wear reflect the things that are hidden deep inside of you. They're a statement about something close to your world. Fashion is a way of turning yourself inside out.
>
> ELISABETH ROHM, ACTOR

All of these locale and media factors influence how people ultimately present themselves to the world.

UNVEILING THE REAL YOU IN YOUR CLOSET

If you collect clothes in your closet without purging every season or two, you possess a Rorschach test that reveals your fashion personality and life history. Spend some time with *you* and "read" what is hanging in your closet and what it says about you. Your clothes have everything to do with your likes and dislikes.

An organized closet may reflect an organized mind and life. However, too much organization kicks up a red flag. For example, do you always hang outfits together? If so, is it because you want to remember you bought them to go together, or because you aren't comfortable wearing the pieces any other way? That doesn't maximize your wardrobe dollars. It can also be a sign you're afraid to take a chance, or you are not comfortable with change or newness. Some women feel insecure about their ability to mix and match their clothes. Then you risk looking the same all the time.

Another common discovery is miniwardrobes in different sizes. Maintaining wardrobes for skinny times, average times, and "fat" times is a waste of money and a constant reminder of your weight and body image issues. Seeing skinny clothes you can't wear is a depressing reminder of your dissatisfaction about what you weigh. Keeping a stash of "fat" clothes discounts confidence about maintaining a weight loss.

A tremendous variance in types of clothes—such as a leather jacket hanging next to five dresses made of delicate lace-trimmed fabrics, bracketed by an assortment of strictly tailored business suits—might reveal a mood dresser. It could also mean you haven't found your true identity or are in a transition. You may be looking for a new self-definition, a new self-concept.

"Your closet represents a collection of your life experiences, attitudes, fears, ambitions, and hopes for the future."

Recognize items in your closet that are "guilt inducers." These are things given to you as presents that you never wear. "I had to get this for you because it looks just like you!" gushes a friend, husband, or your mother-in-law. It is NOT you. It is hideous. But it was expensive, and he or she gave it to you to express love or affection. Savor that thought, take it to a consignment store, and lose the guilt.

Clothes may be markers of special events or indicators of life changes. It is easy to read in a woman's closet when her employer moved from corporate to casual dressing, or her change from living in a city to the suburbs or a resort area.

You'll learn about the tales your closet tells in greater depth in chapter 5, Closetology 101.

YOUR HISTORY IS NOT WHO YOU ARE TODAY

Who are you today? The signs are all there in your closet if you look closely enough. For women this is an exceedingly important exercise, because appearance is a key factor in how society values—or devalues—a woman.

Fortunate women reach a point in their lives when they realize that the really important thing is what's inside them, who they are today. And most often, they have changed their appearance to reflect this wisdom. Feeling confident and connected, inside and outside, is what it's all about.

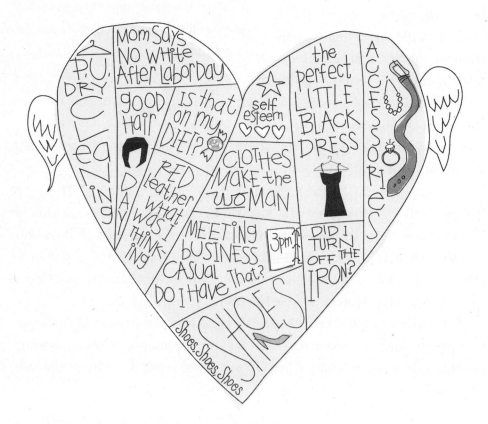

CHAPTER FOUR

DISCOVER YOUR FASHION PERSONA— INTERNAL SELF-EXPRESSION

Since I was a little girl, I've hated any clothes that you couldn't breathe in or that you had to pull over your head. I developed an allergy to zippers. I love clothes that have movement. Everything in my life is about wanting to be free.

DIANE VON FURSTENBERG, DESIGNER

Now we are going to play fashion sleuth. The suspect is you!

You are about to uncover your "modus operandi"—how you go about creating the "you" the world sees each day. Your visual appearance is your fashion persona.

In psychology, *persona* means the personality an individual projects to others; the term derives from the Latin word referring to masks worn by Etruscan actors. An individual's appearance is primarily a projection of who they *want* to be or what impression they want to project, mixed with elements of their authentic self. Your authentic self is the person you are on the inside, the one who gives you permission to leave dishes in the kitchen sink, occasionally skip exercise class, and not count calories in a snack because you ate it standing up. Few people admit their foibles to the world, so they create an external persona more to their liking, one that reflects their best intentions.

Our goal is to hold up a mirror to you, to help you develop an aware-ness of yourself, of who you are. To help you define your fashion persona we will show you how to uncover your outward expressions in clothing, accessories, and other items in your closet. When your inner personality coincides with your outer appearance, you are harmoniously expressing your personal sense of style.

THE SEVEN DOMINANT FASHION PERSONALITIES

There are seven dominant types of fashion personalities. Definitions and explanations of each type follow. However, *most women are a combination of different persona types, because of career choices or personality quirks or due to the different things they do at different times.* This mix is what makes each of us unique and interesting! For example, you may be a conservative classic in your corporate job, yet outdoorsy and athletically inclined on weekends.

Variations may be subtle or extreme. A fashion executive in our acquaintance wears elegant designer clothes all week, then hops on her Harley-Davidson motorcycle on weekends and speeds off decked out in black leather from head to toe. We also know two men, one a senior executive in a major high-tech company and the other a prominent judge, who both don helmets and head off on their motorcycles each weekend. All of these biker-besotted individuals keep their hobby secret from business associates; it's probably safe to assume that most co-workers would find it challenging to reconcile their day-to-day images of these people with their *Easy Rider* sides.

Sometimes people take persona detours. Judie relates: *Cynthia and I met for lunch after not seeing each other for six years. We used to work as buyers in the same department store. "I have to tell you the strangest story about myself," said Cynthia, who had always been a fashion modernist. "After Jim and I moved to Texas, we lived in an area where there were no buying positions for me. I became friendly with two women who owned a trendy boutique. They invited me to join them as an administrative partner, and I accepted. Judie, they bought the absolute wildest clothes for the store: sweaters trimmed in studs and leather patches, hip hugger jeans with torn spots, leather jackets with enormous shoulder trims, and dresses with all manner of swags, shirring, cutouts, and detail. Before long my closet was loaded with the stuff, and I wore it every day. Two years later, we mutually agreed to close the store. After our going-out-of-business sale, I stood in my closet, looking at my clothes and wondering, 'What was I thinking?' None of it was me. That day, I took it all to a consignment store."*

Judie's analysis: Cynthia is a classic example of situational persona. Instead of maintaining her fashion persona and staying true to it, Cynthia tried to adapt to a new persona she wasn't comfortable with. Eventually (and at great expense), she realized it was not expressing her real, inner personal style.

In your own authentic self, you know your personal, and perhaps secret, quirks of behavior, interests, and pursuits. Keys to them are in *your* closet—just like the black leather, helmets, and Harley-Davidson tee shirts stashed in our friend's closets.

So it's time to put on your Sherlock Holmes hat and investigate the traits of each of the seven dominant fashion personas. See if you recognize yourself in one or more.

1. The Classic—Timeless and Conservative

This is the dominant persona among women across the United States.

Even though *The Preppy Handbook* is out of print, she wears blazers, tailored shirts, trousers, suits, knee-length skirts, trouser socks, loafers, and plain pumps.

Leslie, data manager for a large consumer company, earned an M.B.A. last year by enrolling in a special weekend program at her local college campus. "Although my office is business casual, on my twenty-sixth birthday I decided my wardrobe and appearance should be as impressive as my degree," said Leslie. "I traded in my

THE
Classic
WOMAN

khakis and baggy dresses for tailored skirts, shirts, cashmere sweaters, and dresses. I prefer solid colors, knee-length skirts, and conservative looks. I call them modern classics. They are not funky, or sexy, just appropriate."

"Appropriate" may be a defining description for a Classic. Dressing in a classic manner that is unquestionably appropriate is a way for this woman to feel secure and comfortable. In psychological terms, a Classic is a high self-monitor, meaning she modifies her behavior to be consistent with the demands of a given situation. She wants to make a good impression without necessarily soliciting compliments or creating fireworks.

Recent college graduates, career women, many women who work outside the home, CEO wives, and "ladies who lunch" fall into this classification. She is often a sports fan, from soccer leagues to college teams to the NFL. A stalwart in her neighborhood, business, and community, the Classic may be a supporter of the arts, a gardener, a great cook, or play golf or tennis.

Classic women are rarely "shop till you drop" types. Yet they do have their moments—say, when a new specialty shop, mall, or discount store opens nearby. And they love to shop on vacation, but even on these occasions, the Classic keeps a steady-as-she-goes course.

Jessica, a thirty-eight-year-old mom and sales manager for a hotel, said, "My closet is filled with timeless classics. I never veer very far from the middle of the road. In my work I deal with a wide variety of people. One day I may be planning a religious meeting, and the next a convention of rock promoters or dot-com entrepreneurs."

Accessories are her indulgence. "Each season I splurge on shoes, handbags, belts, and jewelry. These are what I use to transform my classics into the present. My classic clothes give me a level of comfort and confidence, while I think my accessories add a flair that makes me feel feminine, distinctive, and finished."

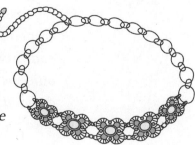

When shopping, Classic women prefer Talbots, Harold's, and Nordstrom, the more understated part of St. John Knits, Josephine Chaus, Ellen Tracy, Dana Buchman, Bill Blass, and Valentino.

2. The Natural—Direct, Unpretentious, Low-Maintenance

The Natural is one of the most ingrained personas. Her look is outdoorsy, clean, unfussy. She is at ease with herself, projecting a breezy yet peaceful demeanor. Often athletically inclined, the Natural woman is in shape. She jogs, walks, plays tennis, hikes, canoes, or kayaks, and may ski. Her hair is likely short and straight or styled into an easy, casual, wash-and-go do. She wears little or no makeup.

Ms. Natural wears seasoned khaki walk shorts or pants, tees, tailored shirts, Polartec, jeans, exercise gear, and serious outdoor sportswear. Her daily uniform may be a white shirt and khakis. The Natural woman is not fond of shopping; she wants to get in, find it, pay for it, and be gone.

Sometimes for a Natural woman like Cynthia, a forty-year-old client, this shopping aversion goes against other instincts. "I have three daughters whose ages range from thirteen to nineteen. Young women are so into fashion today. My daughters' advice and the clothes they pick out for me just don't feel right. I come home from these shopping trips feeling guilty and I emotionally beat up on myself, because mothers are supposed to know about these things and love to go shopping with their daughters," said Cynthia.

"More than anything, I positively dread going to the mall with them. It's so frustrating. I just can't get this creating-a-wardrobe thing right." Her girls used to be compliant shoppers, but when they became teenagers,

things changed. They began urging Cynthia to follow fashion and reach out in the way she dresses.

One fall day during a Southern Women's Show, Cynthia heard Jackie speak on fashion personas. "It was a revelation. I knew instantly I was a Natural. It was pure elation, discovering I did have a sense of style and am not a fashion nightmare," said Cynthia. "I always felt insecure about not knowing how to teach my daughters about selecting clothes for these trendy times. I felt that being a woman, I should know all of this."

In consultations, Jackie helped Cynthia work out a wardrobe plan, and she learned how to mix and match within the framework of her Natural style. Cynthia now has a signature style of her own, and her daughters understand.

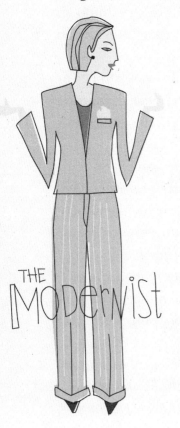

The Natural is a low self-monitor. She is more concerned about her private values than about her surface appearance. Simplicity is a defining trait.

When shopping, the Natural woman prefers Patagonia, L.L. Bean, Title Nine Sports, Sports Unlimited, J. Crew, Tommy Hilfiger, the Gap, and Abercrombie & Fitch.

3. The Modernist—Updated, Sleek, Sophisticated

The Modernist likes things simple, straightforward, and understated in updated modern ways. She is more of an extrovert in style than a Classic: confident, usually social and sophisticated. The Modernist's philosophy is "less is more."

Elegance is restraint.

Many Modernists adopt this uncomplicated style because it is efficient. Urban Modernists may wear suits every day because it helps present them in a way they want others to see them. And they believe suits convey seriousness.

Allison, a corporate marketing executive, says, "I dress in suits or coatdresses simply because I think it projects the image of someone in control, someone confident and conscientious. It also makes getting dressed easier than figuring out what accessories, which shoes, and what handbag to wear. My basic look hasn't varied in years. Well, except for my hemlines moving up or down, or my pants being pleated or flat front, and the silhouette of the legs being wide or narrow."

The Modernist/Classic wears collarless or simple invisible button, envelope-style jackets, pure silk blouses, sleek sweaters and tees, jeans or slim pants with no cuffs, beautiful shoes and understated accessories. She loves stretch fabrics in classical cut shirts and skirts. In her closet is a wardrobe of basic pantsuits, skirts, and jackets in black and perhaps beige or brown. She keeps, or buys repeats, of her understated pieces season after season, as they are choices projecting the assured and elegant appearance that expresses her inner psyche.

Linda calls herself a contemporary/Modernist investor. "Early in my career, a co-worker told me to dress for the position I want, not the one I have. Her advice impressed me when she got promoted before anyone else in our executive trainee class. I buy solid clothes in cream, black, burgundy, or navy—then add colors to change my look, depending upon the occasion. I have to dress professionally as a company manager, but I do add fun elements like a suede or leather jacket or a designer hand-bag."

The look of a Modernist is urbane and simple, with hallmarks of precisely styled hair and makeup. Her handbag is simple and always of fine leather or chic fabric. Her jewelry is real and selected from her collection of favorite pieces.

Marla, president and founder of a real estate development company, says her style is consistent yet constantly evolving. "I buy quality, not quantity. I tend toward clothes with simple, elegant lines in luxury fabrics that are functional and that last. I actually do follow trends, adapting them to my personal style. And I love watching the way my staff dresses—most of them are in their twenties and thirties and they inspire me."

Our Modernist likes to shop and plans purchases carefully, often simply replacing basic functional items from season to season. She'll wear favorite outfits again and again because they are comfortable and make her feel confident that she looks current and right.

At this point, it's all ending the way it started, with simplicity. In the beginning you do simple things because you don't know better. Now you do it because you do know better.

GEOFFREY BEENE, DESIGNER

The Modernist prefers Lauren by Ralph Lauren, Jones New York, Banana Republic, Nicole Miller, Armani, Anne Klein, Elie Tahari, Max Mara, Carolina Herrera, Calvin Klein, and Donna Karan, but not DKNY.

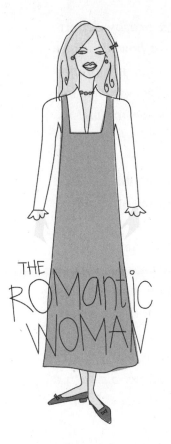

THE ROMANTIC WOMAN

4. The Romantic—Traditional, Nostalgic, Ladylike

The Romantic woman is highly feminine. She wears a single strand of pearls, lace-trimmed slip dresses, pastel colors, tiny stud earrings, small prints, floral motifs, antique jewelry, and loves to shop for special events. She favors long flowing dresses and skirts in both casual and day wear. She loves dainty shoes with tiny straps and delicate heels and has never stopped wearing ballet-style flats or traditional Mary Jane one-strap styles. Her hair may be long, curly, or softly waved. Her nails are always polished and her feet pedicured. Her look is soft, glowing, and all-American.

Historical allusions and cherished notions of the past are powerful influences on this type of woman. She treasures memories of silken hair ribbons, velvet party dresses, and learning to waltz under her father's tutelage or in cotillion dance classes. English country style, classic floral patterns, botanical prints, and delicate details abound both in her home and wardrobe. The Romantic enjoys visiting historic homes and districts. She adores the graceful beauty of calligraphy and of life's ceremonies and celebrations. Each holiday is a fresh opportunity to revisit traditions of the past.

Soft fabrics, pretty flourishes, ruffles, and nostalgically inspired blouses replete with tucking, lace insets, embroidery, and ribbon banding are constants in her closet. Charming Victorian jewelry reproductions catch her eye.

"I am such a hopeless romantic," said Erica, a freelance writer and poet. *"It's funny, how little things give a woman away. Two weeks ago,*

after lunch with three friends, we wandered through a nearby depart-ment store, and I suddenly remembered I needed a velvet bow for a new dinner dress. I said, 'Let's go to Hair Accessories.' Janet, my preppy Boston friend, said, 'Great, I need a new tortoise clip.' Karen, who has ini-tials on everything she owns, said, 'I can check out what's new in Vuitton,' and Tammy, my jogging and kayaking buddy, said, 'What's a hair acces-sory?' "

Many women indulge their Romantic tendencies in decorating their bedrooms, keeping flowers in their homes or office, when selecting a per-sonal fragrance, or in a weakness for scented candles.

A woman with traces of about 10 to 20 percent of Romance in her persona may only express it when dressing for formal occasions, special parties, or weddings. She finds her inner Jane Austen heroine and indulges in softer, prettier clothes than she would feel comfortable select-ing for daytime.

"I love to wear romantic looks after dark," says Marilynn, a mix of ath-letic, classic, and romantic personas. *"It's fun to surprise people with a softer upswept hairstyle, tiny pearls, and gentler styled dresses. I get to show another side of my personality."*

Romantic women adore mother/daughter dressing and outfitting their little boys in Eton short suits or blazers to match Dad. When Judie worked for Storybook Heirlooms catalog for children, the Romantic mom was a target audience. *"The child models are presented as idealized ver-sions of the portrait-perfect little angels mothers imagine or daydream their children to be. The founders came up with their concept while shopping in the children's department of Harrod's, a famed shopping emporium in London."*

When shopping, Ms. Romantic is fond of Jessica McClintock, parts of Betsey Johnson, April Cornell, Ralph Lauren, Lord & Taylor, Eileen Fisher, and Oscar de la Renta. Romantics may also be interested in vintage clothing.

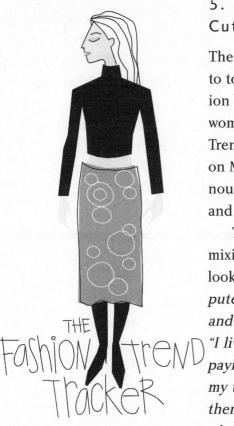

THE Fashion TreND TrackeR

5. Fashion Trend Tracker—on the Cutting Edge

The Trend Trackers' look changes every season, top to toe. They thrive on being the first to sport fashion trends and are risk takers. These self-assured women are high-maintenance, super shoppers. Trend Trackers want to wear the latest looks seen on MTV, in *Elle* or *In Style*. They know how to pronounce *Gucci, Pucci, Givenchy, couturier, faux* and *Tse.*

Trend Trackers are fearless when it comes to mixing colors, textures, fabrics, and prints. They look at doing so as a form of play. *Renee, a computer company sales rep, mixes expensive pieces and discount store finds with a practical abandon. "I live in designer suits but would never dream of paying $300 for a designer-label tee shirt. I buy all my tee shirts at Target," she said, "and when I put them under the jacket of a Calvin Klein pantsuit, who knows?"*

Each fashion season, the minute merchandise starts arriving, they are the first to start buying. If something is hip, or in, they want to wear it. As well as being au courant, Trend Trackers tweak almost everything they wear, giving their clothes an individualistic look.

"I'm totally fashion obsessed," says Sue; "I have been since I was two years old. I've worked in fashion forever in department store display, as a stylist, and now as a party/event planner. I 'style' myself every day when I get dressed. People expect me to look the part of a fashionista."

One day Sue wears vintage clothes, the next she is into a mix of old and new. For her, shopping is entertainment. "I love to wear whatever is the season's hottest look of the moment, and bask in people's reactions. I have my own oddball rules of fashion."

Trend Trackers consider strolling malls and window-shopping creative pastimes. They feel fabrics, scrutinize textures, and appraise outfits on mannequins. Some would rather buy clothes than spend money on food or Broadway show tickets.

"I shop nearly every day," said Kaitlyn, a production assistant. "On my lunch hour or on my way home, I often stop at my favorite specialty store or cruise the mall. I love the way wearing trendy clothes makes me feel. I know I spend too much on clothes, but it's impossible for me to stop."

Trend Trackers know fashion's secret code: the minute hallmarks of a particular designer's work, symbols distinguishing true designer merchandise from knockoffs. They know the names of each season's newest fashion star and how to identify their work.

Along with any kind of fashion business, creative fields such as marketing, the arts, hair salons, and advertising abound with people interested in fashion trends. Walking through these business establishments is like being on a fashion runway. Everyone checks out what everyone else is wearing.

"You can always tell the clients by the safe, classic way they dress," giggles Kaitlyn. "Our clients expect us to know what's hot right now."

Trend Trackers gravitate to designer labels because they are the hot ones of the moment, because certain labels in clothes and accessories have come to signify a certain type of fashion-assured woman.

"I'd be lying if I said I don't care about labels," says Heidi, a public relations ace. "I favor Bill Blass and Oscar de la Renta suits because suits are my work staples and theirs have an updated twist. Suits project a seriously businesslike image at press conferences or meetings. My jewelry is designer—Angela Cummings, Elsa Perretti, David Yurman, Robert Lee Morris. It looks understated but still gets noticed, and I like that."

Trackers populate Bebe, Anthropologie, Forever XXI, Arden B, Max Studio, Savvy Department at Nordstrom, Wet Seal, and Jeffrey. Lines they love include BCBG, INC, and Shelli Segal for Laundry. Seasoned Trackers haunt bridge and designer departments of large stores to buy or scope out new looks. Faves are Michael Kors, Marc Jacobs, and Prada. Then it's off to Target, Wal-Mart; or less expensive stores to find the looks at prices they can afford.

Age looms as a factor for Trend Trackers. Like that old adage "It's hard to be hip and over forty," fashion trends "weed out" women who find other things occupying their minds and lives, or simply whose maturing bodies betray their ability to wear Trend Tracker sizes and styles.

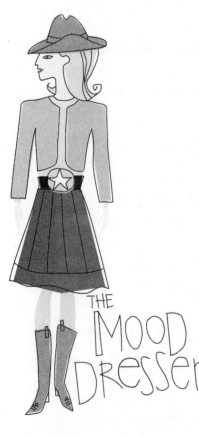

THE MOOD DRESSer

6. Mood Dresser—Bohemian, Creative, Artistic

The Mood Dresser is a chameleon, constantly changing her style. She goes into the world every day dressed as a different persona. *"I do not understand women who lay out the night before what they are going to wear the next day. Forget it. I couldn't possibly do that, because I never know how I'm going to feel in the morning," says Edi, a cosmetic and beauty stylist.*

This Miss has a low threshold for boredom. Her closet bulges, filled with impulsive purchases she may have worn only once or twice. There is an array of clothes some might think could serve as a theater wardrobe. Some ensembles seem inspired by historical literary heroines: poetic, prim, period pieces. Others are soft gauze, flowing, oversize. Clustered together, a black leather miniskirt hangs next to a fringed ankle-length suede skirt and matching fringed vest, green suede jeans, a turquoise leather hooded jacket, and a rawhide shirt sprinkled with turquoise studs. Evening gowns smothered in sequins and beads hang beside a black chiffon shirtwaist-style cocktail dress finished with white collar and cuffs. Who is this person of many personalities?

I try to be true to my spirit, to how I'm feeling. . . . Dressing is a form of expression.

MARISKA HARGITAY, ACTOR

Designer Ralph Lauren once said, "I sell dreams." Mood Dressers dream, and dress for them. She is eclectic and bohemian; one day she is an equestrienne-bedecked city dweller temporarily away from her paddock. The next day she is a country noblewoman in tartan plaids, Shetland sweaters, and a pure cotton shirt. On weekends she turns up in a Navajo-patterned sweater, western boots, and beat-up classic jeans finished with a silver concha belt. By Sunday afternoon she is bounding about in country club tennis whites.

Peeking into the closets of clients who are Mood Dressers presents a dilemma for us. Who is the real persona?

"My closets are mini department stores just full of stuff," exclaims Bette. "I dress for my moods. The problem is, sometimes it takes me hours to decide who I am so I can dress for it."

Judie took a trip into the many moods of Bette. "It's like a carousel of fashion with no rhyme or reason—multiple personalities to the max. To clarify things, we needed to step back and get Bette to reveal her inside reasons for this mode of dressing. Several dramatic shifts in her life had altered her perception of herself. She is in search of herself, not a new outfit."

"At times, it is overwhelming to get dressed to go somewhere," Bette said. "I hate to admit it, but I change clothes a half dozen times before *deciding on an outfit. One time I was literally getting out of my car to go in someplace, when I stopped, drove home, and changed clothes again. I am never sure if I have the right look. At other times, I 'play a part' for the day or occasion."*

Bette emerged with a clearer idea of why she dressed the way she did, and also discovered a surprising love of the organization that emerged from the previous chaos. "It's almost a diagram for my life, yet I haven't sacrificed the sense of fun I get out of dressing up sometimes to suit a mood."

A Mood Dresser likes novelty and selectively chooses fashion trends striking her fancy, often ignoring key looks everyone else latches on to. Artistic license is a hallmark. She's fond of exotic ensembles inspired by foreign countries, or regional American looks such as Southwest, great northern woods, or island-bound Florida tourist. She selects clothes because of the emotions they evoke.

"This black leather pantsuit makes me feel strong, powerful, and sexy. It's this Avengers *thing—undercover agent, international intrigue," says Ines.*

The Mood Dresser may simply try on a different personality each day because it amuses her.

"I like to get up each morning and decide who I am going to be that day, depending on what appointments or events I have on my calendar," says Terra, a writer and teacher. "It's fun to dress a part to back up an article I might be trying to sell to an editor. To pitch a fashion piece over lunch, I wear the latest and go for an edge in my appearance. For a children's magazine, I'm a typical mom in my mom-mobile. For a feature piece on art, I dress in black and wear my most collectible jewelry."

Mood Dressers are likely to have a vast selection of accessories, with jewelry ranging from simple gold hoops or studs to large, multistrand beaded necklaces, carved wood symbols, piles of pearls, plus a collection of original handcrafted necklaces, pins, or bracelets.

Young women experimenting with radically different looks are "trying on" different versions of themselves. It's a way of working out discrepancies between their real self and an ideal self based on a passing fancy or pop idol. Until she discovers who she is, the process involves changes in looks, clothes, and even behaviors.

Artistic and bohemian women are Mood Dressers because they view getting dressed as one more opportunity for creativity. They are into yoga, peasant blouses, ethnic looks, unusual jewelry, and scented candles. A few decades ago, these women would be dubbed "hippies." Such women eschew fashion formulas in favor of self-expression. *Anna, a San Francisco–based artist, favors looks she says are "slightly off-kilter, not at all fashiony. I really love to mix odd colors, most artists do. And I like unexpected elements mixed: a sweeping taffeta skirt worn with a sweater and some offbeat footwear."*

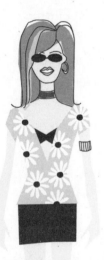

Delilane, a news photographer in Washington, says she wears rugged clothes in her work "because I am in and out of my car all day in heat, rain, humidity, and dust. But on my own time, I truly believe fashion is a language describing to people who you are. I'm not interested in trendy fashion, but sometimes something comes along and I have to have it. In my work I notice what people wear, and almost always it tells me something about their personality or interests."

From flea markets to vintage stores, mall chains to the Salvation Army, Mood Dressers are insatiable shoppers.

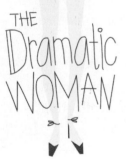

7. Dramatic Women—Ready for Their Close-up

Dramatic women fall into several subcategories. Ignoring all fashion trends, each woman in these subcategories has her own vision of how she wants to look.

Often confused with Trend Trackers, **entrance makers** are Dramatic women intent on telling the world how au courant and wonderful they are. They *expect* compliments each time they grace an event. Super self-monitors, Dramatic women are extremely concerned about how they appear in public. They spend hours putting together the perfect eye-catching outfit for each major occasion. Entrance makers wear attention-getting and often extremely expensive jewelry, bright colors or arresting printed fabrics, freshly detailed hairstyles, elaborate makeup, drop-dead hats, handbags, and shoes. They have a weakness for fur coats and jackets, feathers and trailing shawls.

"Helene's closet looks like a rainbow," reports a close friend. "Everything is arranged by color . . . and what colors! Her jewelry is placed on velvet in thin drawers covered with Plexiglas. Individual plastic box drawers stacked to the ceiling are filled with shoes. Her belts are on one of those rotating tie racks designed to hold a hundred selections. She has pocket silks and lace hankies, a virtual bouquet of artificial flower pins, gloves, and dozens of silk scarves."

Being a Dramatic entrance maker requires a major time commitment, what with planning, shopping, coordination, and execution. Her payoff is the emotional satisfaction she receives from others' adulation and admiration.

Entrance makers are in the front row at fashion and trunk shows. They demand exclusivity and assurance that no one else in their geographic area will be sold a duplicate.

Logo ladies are Dramatic women who build their confidence and self-esteem by wearing clothing and accessories imprinted with designer logos. These women are comforted by their belief that designer logos indicate good taste, quality, and great expense.

Bobbi projects her chic, sexy style through

accessories. *"I pride myself on being the best-dressed woman in the room. My must-have is a designer handbag and shoes. Wearing designer merchandise tells people I recognize the best and deserve it."*

Collecting clothes and accessories with designer logos is an expensive way of dressing. Or more commonly, it requires a certain amount of subterfuge locating credible knockoffs or cheap copies of designer goods, which are then used to fool friends or the world at large.

Some designers, charging stratospheric prices for their merchandise, understand this customer in a diabolical way. It has been suggested they deliberately put their logo on outrageous and tasteless designs to see just how far these gullible consumers will go in their search for status. Nearly every season, these designers prove themselves correct and laugh all the way to the bank.

Occasionally an item with a logo becomes a must-have status purchase. Its powerful appeal sweeps even conservative and clear-thinking women along in its wake and out of their regular personas. Frequently the expensive item is a handbag emblazoned with designer initials or an obvious tag/label with a designer name on it. Leather, suede, and especially fur have special élan because most scream "I am expensive" and people know it. Logo ladies love the gratification they receive by owning items broadcasting their fashion savvy and "I'm worth it" expense.

It becomes a case of not *what* you wear but *who* you wear that defines you.

At a holiday party this year, the hostess directed Jackie to the guest room where guests put their coats and handbags. She was struck by the array of designer logo bags on the bed, all shapes and sizes, each bearing a designer's initials or full name. Six were identical, not exactly a statement for their owner's originality. It can be a way of announcing, "I belong to this income group because I can afford this bauble."

Logo ladies shop at Neiman Marcus, Saks, Henri Bendel, Bergdorf's and company-owned designer boutiques such as Escada, Versace, Burberry, St. John and Ralph Lauren.

Geography plays a role in ***cultural dramatic dressers.*** For example, Texas Head Turners have their own traditional mores of dressing, including big fluffy-styled hair, western boots (occasionally with evening clothes), and top-to-toe coordination; i.e., turquoise hair clips to match their turquoise shoes. She *never* goes to the grocery store unless she is turned out in full hair and makeup. And she is extremely sensitive to Texas men's opinions about her appearance. Texas women have historical affinities for turquoise and silver jewelry, jeans and denim, broomstick skirts, cowboy shirts and hats.

In the great Southwest, women love the atmosphere, history, colors, and lore of the territory and delight in dressing in ways inspired by traditions. They dress to express their sense of connection. Though demonstrative, you could also say this tendency is romantic. Their challenge comes when they travel or move to other parts of the country, where residents might not understand their motives and consider such ensembles to be almost costumes.

Several types of dramatic appearance defy classification. For example, there are the freeze-dried dolls, ***women "stuck in time."*** These women decided at some point in their past (perhaps when they were cheerleaders, beauty contest finalists, or homecoming queens) that they had reached their most attractive self and vowed never to change a thing. Sure tip-offs are teased hair or odd, brightly colored makeup. If you have been wearing the same hairstyle for more than five years, it could be a tip-off. You might want to consider a subtle or dramatic change.

A variation is the woman who sticks with an old look yet keeps adding to it, unaware that it has become dramatically weird or overdone, as well as inappropriate for her age. Her makeup selections are the same this year as six or seven years ago. This type may need to consider a modern makeover if she has difficulty finding her usual foundation or lipstick color.

The vamp is a Dramatic with an image of herself as a slinky, seductive siren. She projects a sexy persona with clothing, hair, makeup, and a demeanor accessorized by an undulating, practiced walk. Her traits are so fixed that costume designers for films and television manipulate the dress of fictional characters to indicate her personality type.

Julia Roberts's Oscar-winning portrayal of Erin Brockovich certainly owed partial credit to her scanty, tight-fitting wardrobe and exposed bras. The vamp loves animal prints and blouses unbuttoned down to there. Her skirts are short, her hair is long, her pants are tight, and her breasts are up and at 'em. This gal has worn black lace since she was twelve and a half years old. Her breasts may not be original equipment, and chances are she has a collection of "wonder bras."

The vamp shops at Cache, Lillie Rubin, and Bebe.

A CAUTION

Guessing another person's persona can be a slippery slope, so don't turn it into a parlor game. After reading or hearing these descriptions, most women know in their deepest being exactly what fashion persona or mix of personas they possess. Woe be unto friends who tell them, "I'm sure you are a _____."

People can become testy when identified incorrectly, and the lines between personas get fuzzy due to your own perceptions. For example: are color choices expressive of a persona? Some color selections such as mauve or slate could be tagged Modernist—while plum or peach qualifies as a Trend-Tracking "color" of the current season. Neutral color preferences seem Classic, yet black-clad city dwellers see their choice as sophisticated.

For reasons of self-image many women cling to a persona, when in fact due to age, geographic relocation, a new job, or life change, they are in transition or have morphed into a new combination of personas.

THE ROLE OF FASHION TRENDS
IN PERSONA

Every type of fashion persona is influenced by fashion trends. Trends are not always one-season phenomena. Generally they move through our culture over a period of two or three years, then vanish; or else they remain, becoming a long-term force.

Occasionally a fashion trend starts out as a "look of the season" then continues reappearing because of consumer acceptance until it becomes a so-called new classic. When animal prints first burst into fashion they were confined to jungle cat prints. The next season brought on zebra stripes, then cow prints and antelope patterns. All found favor, and over a period of about five years, animal prints became a consistent fashion category and influenced home fabrics, linens, and furniture, culminating in an Ernest Hemingway collection.

Classic personas are moved by trends with intensely personal appeal such as color, or trends that gain acceptability through design refinement. In the late 1990s, pleated pants for women prevailed in classic areas. Then came flat-front styles with side or back zippers. At first Classics were uncomfortable with the figure-revealing silhouette of flat-front pants, until they were shown the style made them look *thinner*. Classics eagerly embraced the style, discovering that sweaters worn outside these trim pants gave coverage and a narrower profile.

Naturals might seem to be impervious to trends. Not so. Athletic shoes are a reference, as season after season shoe designers tout new aerodynamic designs with air bubble inserts and different color combinations and materials. Athletic gear is constantly changing, reflecting new fabric properties, color trends, and even names of rising and falling sports heroes.

How you respond to a fashion trend is an integral part of your fashion persona. The quicker you try a new look, the more of a risk taker or Trend Tracker you may be. Trend Trackers and some Dramatics are early adapters, people who want to separate themselves from the pack, express their adventurous streak, stand out.

Women who accept fashion trends after exposure in magazines, on television, and in stores do so because the trends have been absorbed through repetition, then refined or repackaged by designers or manufacturers, making them more easily acceptable and understood.

THE BELL CURVE OF FASHION TRENDS

Fashion trends move like a bell curve. Remember bell curves? Those charts high school and college teachers use for distributing class grades? Demographers chart things like income, diseases, and socioeconomic trends on bell curves. Trends start small in discovery mode, slowly grow through exposure, bloom, and peak, before falling and dwindling off the chart.

Merchandisers have used fashion bell curves for decades as an instrument for classifying customers and predicting their purchasing plans. In the discovery phase, first they test a trend. If it creates positive customer reaction, stock is increased during the growth and peak stages, when the look finds wide acceptance. As a look declines, merchants stock less expensive and classically modified versions until the trend disappears from fashion's radar.

The different fashion personas consistently fall into a specific acceptance place on a graph from discovery, growth, peak, and the downside decline of a fashion trend. The arc of fashion trends is emotionally revealing, and not only on an individual level. The bell curve arc of a fashion trend is also a study in human behavior and adaptation, a key field in psychology.

Fashion Trackers are *early adapters,* the first to seize trends in discovery. Mood Dressers and certain Dramatic types, such as creative or status-seeking women, dabble next in new fashion ideas. The Mood Dresser may be a Tracker if a trend is exotic, such as peasant dressing. Modernists, by their nature, are aware and receptive at this point. Later, Romantics and

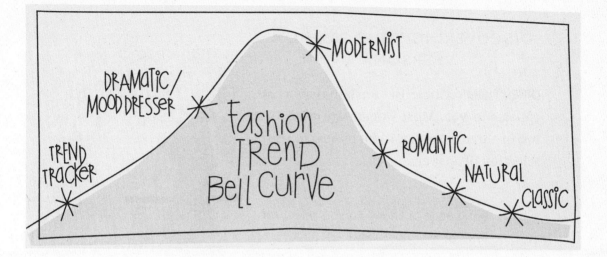

Naturalists pick and choose among trends they might find interesting or agreeable to their fashion persona. The Natural may be a Tracker if the trend involves athletic clothing or shoes. The Natural may also be an extremely late adapter of one-year trend cycles, or may not participate at all. By peak time most of the personas have sampled or are aware of trends, but Classics are usually the last to tap in and become consumers.

Minitrends also occur within individual personas. For example, logo ladies tend to migrate from logo to logo as designers emerge, flame, and attain must-have status. An example is Kate Spade, a designer who hit with minimalist handbags in the 1990s. Younger women immediately dropped their former status bags and flocked to Kate's fresh new silhouettes. But consumers eventually get bored and want to move on to the next hot symbol with stylish cache.

Think about yourself. What was the last fashion trend you tried, and when did you try it? Where would you place yourself on a fashion trend arc?

Now that you understand the characteristics of different fashion personas, move on and take this quiz to discover your personal persona or mix of personas!

DISCOVERING YOUR FASHION PERSONA

DIRECTIONS: Circle the answer that most appeals to you. Most women are a mix of two or three personas, so be honest in your selection of answers.

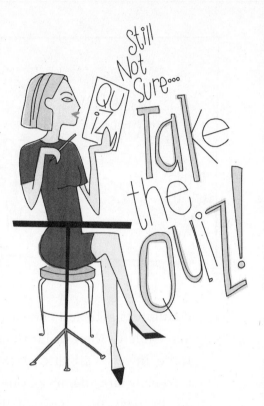

1. What style of shoes do you select for work or everyday wear?
   a. I like a low-heel pump for work. I have one style in several basic colors.
   b. I buy a pair to match every outfit for work or play. I prefer flat heels, and if it has a bow, I have to have it!
   c. Shoes are my passion! The higher the heel the better! I go shoe shopping every season and love new trends. My latest purchase is a pair of suede boots.
   d. There are lots of shoes in my closet, lots of different styles. I have a hard time figuring out what to put with what.

2. What is your favorite shoe for evening wear, special occasions, or formal attire?
   a. I prefer an elegant yet simple higher heel.
   b. My dressy shoe is a black silk pump with a midheel. It is comfortable and goes with everything.
   c. Silver and gold heels are my staple. I like a sexy look to complete my outfit.
   d. My lifestyle doesn't lend itself to needing a dressy shoe.

3. What is your favorite piece of jewelry?
    a. I treasure the cultured pearls I received as a birthday gift. I wear them all the time. They are one strand and layer at my neckline.
    b. My wedding band. It is simple and elegant. It is the only piece of jewelry I wear, except for pierced stud earrings.
    c. I have lots of fashion jewelry. I like colored pieces that go with each outfit in my wardrobe.
    d. Simple architectural pieces like large pins, pendants, and earrings.

4. Select your first choice for earrings.
    a. Small- or medium-size hoops in gold or silver. I only wear "real" jewelry and usually the same pieces every day.
    b. I am allergic to the nickel in costume earrings. I like a 14-karat gold ball earring.
    c. I don't have a favorite. I have to see what matches the outfit I select each day or evening.
    d. Whatever is in for the season.

5. How would you describe your makeup appearance?
    a. My shades are soft with a slight touch of eye color.
    b. I like a bold look. Bright lip colors and false eyelashes are a staple.
    c. I have drawers full of makeup and often change my look.
    d. I wear very little makeup. Lipstick and a little mascara, and I am out the door.

6. What colors do you favor in nail polish? Toenail polish?
    a. I love to shop for nail color. Right now I am into deep, dark colors.
    b. My nails are usually done in a French manicure or just a little clear polish.

    c. I purchase lots of different colors and never wear any of them.

    d. Pale pink, or a soft coral on my nails. On my toes, the same color darker.

7. What do you prefer to sleep in at night?
    a. Tee shirts and boxer shorts. Comfy and simple.
    b. My favorite is a floral long gown and matching robe in flannel or cotton.
    c. I like a silk slithery gown with a little touch of lace and matching peignoir.
    d. Nothing!

8. What is your favorite piece of lingerie?
    a. I like short silk gowns at times and sometimes a soft cotton oversize tee shirt.
    b. My lacey red bustier and a matching thong.
    c. My cotton pajama set or a simple long gown.
    d. My Victorian-style bastiste gown with tucks and lace.

9. How do you select a handbag?
    a. It's got to be functional. I like compartments and ease.
    b. I look for the designer brands first and then look at style.
    c. I buy quality in a neutral color and use one basic handbag for a long time.
    d. Casual cloth and crochet bags are a favorite.

10. How often do you purchase a handbag?
    a. I purchase two fine leather bags a season.
    b. Every chance I get. I love the coolest bags in a variety of colors, sizes, and shapes.
    c. I purchase similar bags in different colors for choice.
    d. When my handbag wears out.

11. Do you like a variety of color in your wardrobe?
    a. Yes! The brighter the better.
    b. I buy what I like and I always look at the color of the season.
    c. Black! Black! Black is my color!
    d. I like color, but I don't know how to accessorize it.

12. Do you like patterns or solid fabrics?
    a. Exotic prints, batiks, and rough textures.
    b. I prefer solids. If I wear a pattern, it might be a stripe or dot.
    c. Small florals attract me. I also like a muted stripe.
    d. I like to mix patterns and colors for a different look. I love big prints.

13. Pick the type of sweater you might purchase.
    a. Body conscious. Bright color with appliqué or pattern.
    b. Turtlenecks in all colors. Same style, various fabrics. Oversize or regular.
    c. Twin sweater sets in basic colors.
    d. All different types, colors, and styles.

14. Do you prefer a cardigan sweater or a jacket as your third piece?
    a. I like the look of a jacket. Jackets and pantsuits are a staple in my lifestyle.
    b. I love soft cardigans that go with my longer skirts and make an outfit.
    c. Each season, I look over my prior season jackets and sweaters. This classification is important to me. I like to purchase something new in both areas to update my wardrobe.
    d. I like to emulate what is in the magazines or on display at the stores.

15. You've received a gift. Which one of the following selections would make you smile?
    a. A pale pink cardigan sweater.
    b. A 14-karat gold bangle bracelet.
    c. Unusual handcrafted one-of-a-kind jewelry.
    d. Subscriptions to fashion magazines.

16. Have you ever received a gift that was "not you?" Select one of the options that describe it or are similar.
    a. Yes! A pair of brown leather jeans. I never wear leather.
    b. If I don't like it, I return it.
    c. A gift certificate from one of those classic stores. Ugh! I purchased a white tee and took the rest in cash.
    d. I like everything I receive and eventually use it.

17. Select the cocktail look you would choose for a special night out.
    a. I buy dressy separates and pull them together, depending on the occasion.
    b. A strapless multicolored sequined short dress.
    c. Black satin trousers with a beaded jacket and shell.
    d. A cream lace dress and jacket.

18. Describe how you want to look for a dressy occasion.
    a. Different from anyone else.
    b. In the newest style for the season.
    c. Understated in a chic black dress or separates in a beautiful fabric.
    d. I wear my one dressy silk suit. It goes anywhere.

19. Select the types of fabrics or patterns you like to wear.
    a. I like a lot of different fabrics and patterns mixed together.
    b. I don't like patterns. I prefer solids.
    c. I only wear natural fibers. My patterns are always florals in muted shades.
    d. I prefer luxurious fabrics . . . silks, wool, cashmere, and fine cottons.

20. Describe your favorite style of swimsuit.
    a. A tank suit! Something I can swim in.
    b. Bikini in a bright color or an unusual one-piece style.
    c. It depends on my weight. I have many different styles.
    d. None! I won't wear one.

21. Select the type of everyday china or fine china you would prefer.
    a. A basic white set for every day.
    b. A set with architectural shapes in solid colors.
    c. My china is eclectic. Lots of different styles mixed together.
    d. I like a set with muted small flowers or a blue and white pattern.

22. What type of silverware might you select?
    a. An intricate gold ware set.
    b. A sculptural set in matte finish.
    c. I have an inexpensive set I purchased at a discount store.
    d. I use the set my mom gave me. It's okay.

23. Select a bed covering that most appeals to you.
    a. Denim covers with matching pillows.
    b. Eyelet covers with matching pillows.
    c. Solid duvet with different pillows for every season.
    d. Animal print with lots of tapestry pillows.

24. Do you like to wear designer logos on your clothing or accessories?
    a. Sometimes I do. It depends on where I am going and the occasion.
    b. I do not like any logos anywhere on or near my body.
    c. I may do that in an understated handbag.
    d. Yes, I do! I know they are the finest quality.

25. Select your favorite type of hosiery.
    a. I like trouser socks. I always wear trousers.
    b. A neutral pair of hose. I never wear colors on my legs.

    c. I have lots of choices. Fishnet, stripes, colors where they match.

    d. I may or may not wear hose, depending on the outfit.

26. Describe your favorite style of sofa.
    a. Lots of cushions with a botanical or floral covering.
    b. Simple leather with a nail head trim.
    c. Solid fabric and a variety of throw pillows so I can change them with the seasons.
    d. Antique sofa with needlepoint covering.

27. Describe your ideal coat (if money were no object).
    a. One that is warm!
    b. A black trench coat.
    c. A long double-breasted camel hair coat is my choice.
    d. A long fur coat.

28. Describe the type of gloves you might purchase.
    a. Leather gloves in bright colors.
    b. Black knit gloves.
    c. Black leather gloves.
    d. A famous designer plaid.

29. Select the watchband you prefer.
    a. A silver and gold metal band mixed together.
    b. My choice is a black leather strap.
    c. A gold designer watch with rhinestone trim.
    d. I like a fashion watch with interchangeable colored straps.

30. Describe your favorite hairstyle.
    a. I change my style with the season.
    b. Short and easy.
    c. Long and curly with a headband.
    d. A shoulder-length sleek and simple cut.

DIRECTIONS: In the key below, circle the letter next to the A,B,C, or D you circled for each question. For example: on question 2 if you chose B, you would circle F. For question 3 if you chose C, you circle G. Do the same until you have circled a letter for each of the thirty questions.

Many women know their type immediately. Most, however, are mixes of several types, with one being dominant. For example, your score may look like this: 11 E scores, 9 C scores, 8 D scores, and 2 A scores indicates a mix of Modernist, Trend Tracker, and Dramatic.

1. A-A	2. A-E	3. A-B	4. A-A	5. A-B
B-B	B-F	B-F	B-H	B-G
C-C	C-G	C-G	C-D	C-D
D-D	D-H	D-E	D-C	D-F

6. A-C	7. A-B	8. A-D	9. A-F	10. A-E
B-E	B-F	B-C	B-C	B-G
C-D	C-E	C-F	C-A	C-D
D-B	D-G	D-B	D-B	D-H

11. A-G	12. A-D	13. A-G	14. A-E	15. A-B
B-D	B-A	B-F	B-B	B-E
C-E	C-B	C-A	C-H	C-D
D-F	D-C	D-D	D-C	D-C

16. A-A	17. A-E	18. A-D	19. A-C	20. A-A
B-H	B-G	B-C	B-A	B-G
C-G	C-A	C-E	C-B	C-D
D-D	D-B	D-F	D-E	D-H

21. A-A	22. A-G	23. A-H	24. A-C	25. A-A
B-E	B-C	B-C	B-F	B-B
C-D	C-F	C-F	C-A	C-G
D-B	D-H	D-G	D-G	D-F

26. A-A	27. A-F	28. A-C	29. A-A	30. A-C
B-E	B-A	B-A	B-E	B-F
C-D	C-E	C-E	C-G	C-B
D-B	D-G	D-G	D-C	D-A

Tally your score by noting how many times your choices indicate:

A_____ B_____ C_____ D_____

E_____ F_____ G_____ H—no value

The following is the key to the different types.

       A is Classic   E is Modernist

       B is Romantic   F is Natural

       C is Trend Tracker   G is Dramatic

       D is Mood Dresser   H no value

The higher the score by each letter, the stronger the indication of your fashion persona. Your total should equal 30.

CHAPTER FIVE

CLOSETOLOGY 101: A BLUEPRINT TO CLEAR THE CHAOS AND ESTABLISH ORDER

My closet looks like a convention of multiple personality cases.

ANNA QUINDLEN, AUTHOR

Everybody has something to hide, and it is usually his or her closet. Most are a shambles—cramped, crowded, and packed full of clutter. It is embarrassing! You bring it on yourself, and you know it. That unruly pile living in your closet is the product of a lot of thought, effort, and expense. It is a mess, but it's *your* mess. And yes, we understand, you've been meaning to clean out that closet for months.

Clients confess to shuffling Jackie's business card around their desk for as long as a year before they call for an appointment. "I had it on my bulletin board for eight months," says Carla. "Every look at it soothed my conscience, because I knew one day I would pick up the phone and ask her to come gut the scariest room in *my house—my closet. Rather than try to sort it out, I always went out and just bought something new. My closet is just out of control. Finally I did it."*

Our analysis: a cluttered closet is a monument to delusional thinking and a symptom of cognitive dissonance. It's a mess right there in front of your eyes, yet you refuse to acknowledge it because in your stress-battered life, you don't want to see it. It bugs you, yet you carefully selected, collected, and paid for everything in there. *The variety of stuff in your closet is uniquely you. Each item is indicative of a state of mind experienced by you at some point, because you choose to keep it.* The man in your life might choose to keep a skateboard or a boat anchor long after he can use it. That's his kind of stash. He thinks he might use those things again someday. Your personal kind of clutter, say a pair of four-inch red stiletto-heeled sandals and a feather boa, is quite different. You keep those things because you *want* them. And you have a deeply ingrained reason.

Closets are supposed to be a place to store the clothes, accessories, and shoes you wear. Many that we see look like archeological digs, filled with layers of stuff from days past. Others are more selective; they remind us of scrapbooks documenting a woman's life: there's the dress she wore when she got engaged, her wedding dress, the pantsuit she wore a wondrous day in Paris, the gown from her son's bar mitzvah, the only size 4 suit she could ever fit into, and her daughter's prom dress.

Other closets, frankly, can only be classified as bottomless pits. The specter of what you might find on the bottom is scary.

My closet is divided into three sections—Normally Overweight, Seriously Overweight, and Never Been That Thin. I do not like to think about the amount of money I have wasted on clothes I just needed to lose a few more pounds to wear.

MOLLY IVINS, AUTHOR

You accumulate and hold on to all that stuff in your closet because of emotions, past attachments, or present challenges.

"There are clothes everywhere, and she says she has nothing to wear," sputtered one husband to Jackie. *"My wife has taken over every closet in the house. You've got to help her."*

He—not his wife—had hired me. When I arrived at their home, there were not only closets full of unworn clothing, but also bags everywhere full of ticketed, never-before-worn purchases. As we chatted, I asked Ellie what her goal was for our time together. "I want to get down to one closet, so I can really see what I have to work with to get dressed," she said. We plunged ahead, examining every piece in each closet.

We began to compile the clothes we would eventually reject, and we broke these "reject" clothes into categories: (1) what we could return to stores for credit; (2) what we could take to a consignment shop and get some money back for; and (3) what we could donate to a women's resource center for its "job interview closet." (This last category converted problems into pluses by providing a positive way to help less fortunate women.)

The closetology process focused Ellie's thinking. She was amazed at how often she had been rebuying the same things. She actually had four identical skirts, all unworn. At the same time, she began to realize how her closet chaos had originated. "I just haven't been thinking clearly," she admitted. "I've simply been shopping out of boredom. I never thought about how much money I was spending until I saw it today, in front of me. It's a sobering experience."

The process helped Ellie zero in on why she was using shopping as a substitute for what she really wanted in her life. She confessed she had been trying to get pregnant for years. Her constant shopping was an outlet for her unhappiness. After our time together, Ellie approached her husband about adopting a baby, and they started the process. Several months later, as often happens, Ellie became pregnant. Today she has three children and shares one closet with her happy husband.

Soon after Judie met Becky, a successful advertising executive in San Francisco, Becky boldly spoke about her closets full of clothes: *"I have three houses—one in the city, our weekend place, and one at the beach . . . all of my closets at each are stuffed." This statement reveals that Becky is someone with substantial assets and lots of possessions. It makes Becky feel rich to have all that stuff. It's emotionally comforting, because as a child she wore hand-me-down clothes and her family could never afford to own a house of their own. "We moved a lot . . . to about eight different cities before I was in the tenth grade. My childhood was pretty chaotic. It never seemed like I belonged anywhere."*

FEAR, POTENTIAL, AND THE MEMORIES IN YOUR CLOSET

Fear of loss prevents many women from purging their closets, especially women who've experienced dramatic changes in their personal life. *Five years after a traumatic divorce, Candace's closet spills over with once-expensive clothes. "I'm afraid I'll never be able to have things like these again," she said.*

The reasons you collect valuable goodies in your closet may be less clear. Sometimes they embody potential things you want to do or be. Sparkly cocktail dresses hang ready to go out for a glamorous evening, while ski pants, a matching jacket, leather ski gloves, and long underwear link you to your yearning to return to the mountains of Colorado after one trip many years ago. You may see potential in hoarding things you believe will "come back." Rainbow-colored platform shoes? Neon lime green hip huggers? Fringed leather? Leg warmers? Do we want those things to come back?

We've often heard women on shopping trips say, "This suit will be perfect for a luncheon at the club," when in reality they never allow themselves the luxury of a leisurely luncheon with friends outside of the office. The wife of a corporate executive plops an op art–style, sequin-sprinkled tee shirt on the counter, saying "This is so much fun. I can wear it club-hopping." Few of these items are ever likely to be worn to those destinations—but they give you the *potential* to be ready, just in case.

Sara Jane's closet is filled with exquisite designer suits, leftovers from her business career. She's a forty-two-year-old, stay-at-home mom now, but those suits make her feel important because of what she used to do. They reassure her. It's a phony stage prop she doesn't need, because her life is filled with new important things to do—raising a family. Different things mean different things to different people.

Go to your closet and look inside. What are the emotional reasons you hoard stuff? Memories? Potential? Ego boosting? Fear? Aspirations? Comfort? We each spin our web of reasons, yet when you look in the closet of your best friend, what do you see? Stuff! An aged dress sagging on a worn satin hanger, a tiny leather mini-skirt with the price ticket attached, faded sport clothes, a dented straw hat embellished with dusty flowers, outdated fashion items. To your friend they seem valuable, just like the clutter in your closet seems to be valuable to you. Yet in the final analysis, your clutter and hers are just stuff: old clothes, outdated shoes, stretched-out pants, and worn-out athletic gear. It serves no purpose in your day-to-day life. That old stuff is your past. The future is now, today, bubbling with shining possibilities.

"Our aim is to help you see yourself differently—not as you were yesterday, but as who you are today."

Think you're still not ready to tackle the untamed beast? You need to be ready, not resistant. To ease you into the proper mood, review the following questions.

CLOSET INSIGHT QUIZ

1. It's July. Did you have to flip past wool skirts, tweed jackets, and a flannel vest to get to your favorite white Bermudas? Or it's December. Why is your sundress hanging next to your ski pants? Is that your swimsuit and flowered visor on the closet shelf?

2. Is there a "shrinkage" epidemic taking place in your closet? How many items hanging in there are too tight for you to wear today? Come on—be honest!

3. How often do you wear items residing in your closet such as the plaid skirt with a big gold safety pin, hot pink miniskirt, faux leather motorcycle jacket, or hot pants?

4. Can you wager a guess on how many missing buttons, broken zippers, or permanent stains you could find in your closet?

5. Do you have a "retirement plan" for those stretched-out, faded, exhausted-looking, once-I-loved-them old favorites?

6. Can you tally up the number of unworn "gifts" from well-meaning family or friends you have stashed in there?

7. Do you dare to use a calculator and total up the money you wasted on those items still bearing price tickets and never worn?

8. Can you carry all your shoes needing repairs out to the car in one trip?

9. Is everything hanging in your closet really "you"?

10. If a wardrobe "regular" got lost at the dry cleaners, how long would it take you to miss it?

11. What is the highest number of items you've got on one hanger?

12. How many birthdays have the belts on your belt rack cele-brated? When was the last time you really saw all of them?

13. How much money and how many tubes of lipstick would you find if you went through each and every handbag in there?

14. How long does it take you to find the pair of shoes you need for a specific outfit? Weren't you on your hands and knees groping in dark corners trying to find a matching pair last weekend?

15. How many times have you said, "I really need to clean out my closet"?

GETTING IN THE MIND-SET

Now we hope you are ready! Be brave. Be objective. Get a big glass of ice water. Assemble a notepad and pen, a supply of empty boxes, labels, tape, a Magic Marker, and plastic garbage bags.

If you have a traditional closet with just one door opening onto a larger room, or many small closets in your home, start by taking future-season and past-season garments out of the most convenient space and putting them in another room to be reviewed at the start of the appropri-ate season.

The next step is removing all those tangles of pesky empty wire hang-ers. If you don't have a supply of uniform hangers such as plastic or wood with swivel tops, start collecting them. It is an investment, but if you pick up one or two packages every few weeks you'll soon have a closetful. For pants and skirts we suggest hangers with clips, so you can hang pants and skirts from their waistbands. Folding pants over hangers takes up twice as much room and you end up wearing bump wrinkles at your knees or doing last-minute ironing. Arrange all clothes so they face the same direc-tion. Only one piece per hanger!

For maximum efficiency, keep the current season's clothes in the prime part of your closet. Things you wear the most are best kept front and center. Store out-of-season items in another closet, box, or room. Several companies make slim, big boxes designed to slip under beds for storage. Genius!

Heavy jackets, raincoats, and winter coats belong in the coat/hall closet, along with umbrellas and boots.

Before you start sorting, establish definite destinations: things for charity, things for consignment, and items beyond redemption (otherwise known as trash). Three sisters in Pennsylvania and a group of similar-size girlfriends in Danville, Ohio, have seasonal "swap parties." You might want to add a "swap box" if the idea appeals to you. Anything you haven't worn in the past two years should go into one of these four boxes.

Keep in mind: charitable donations must be genuinely usable. Items destined for consignment or pass-along must be in excellent condition. Ask yourself, "Would I be embarrassed to give this to my best friend?"

Establish a spot for clothes needing repair or alteration, and another stack destined for the dry cleaners.

SEPARATION ANXIETY

Jackie finds that a key role she plays when working with clients as they attack stuffed closets is serving as permission giver. "Hold my hand and give me permission to give this coat to charity. It cost a fortune, but somehow I never wear it that much," said Clarisse.

Be your own permission giver. It's okay for you to get rid of useless or inappropriate things other people gave you as gifts. You are never going to get back the money you invested in that expensive coat you barely wore, but you can free yourself of guilt by removing it from your life. It was a mistake. Get past it.

If you pull a skirt, pants, or blouse out of the closet, and as you look at it immediately have a vague notion that something is wrong with it—a stain, a tear, poor fit—take that thought as a red flag. Find the blemish and decide whether to fix it or pitch it. If you are undecided about a piece, tag it and keep it for a week, then look at it again. This is not a do-or-die process.

SOMEDAY CLOTHES, YOUR NOSTALGIA CORNER, MARKDOWN MISTAKES, AND OTHERS

As you take each piece out of your closet, interview it. Why are you here? How do I feel about you? Are you lively, limp, or over the hill? Is your style classic or current? Do you fit and flatter me? Are you a "someday" piece, a markdown mistake, a nostalgic memento?

Someday Clothes are guilt inducers and reminders of your procrastination. "Someday I will wear this when I lose eight pounds." "Someday I will wear this when it comes back in style." "Someday I may need this again when I gain weight." "Someday I will wear this when I find something to match it." Scrutinize these things carefully. You'll realize most belong in consignment or charity.

And what's going on with all those clothes still bearing price tickets? We'll bet those are your Markdown Mistakes. Put them all in one spot, because there is a serious emotional and financial lesson to be learned from them. Study the ticketed items and ask yourself, "Why did I purchase this?" The answer could be as simple as, "It was an incredible buy, on sale for 75 percent off." Yet if you never wear it, the item represents money wasted. Or "It seemed like the perfect dress for _____." But that fill-in-the-blank event never happened. More money wasted. Get your pocket calculator and tally up a total of the prices you paid for those ticketed, never-worn clothes. It's pretty scary, right? Can you afford to waste that kind of money? Next time you are tempted by an incredible buy or a perfect something you may never wear, think about it. If you make your inner psyche aware of this vulnerability then the next time temptation flares, your brain will send up a caution flag.

Your Nostalgia collection is made up of "story" pieces. One is the dress you wore when you got engaged, or when your son got married. There is your daughter's prom dress or your dad's monogrammed bathrobe. Pack these carefully in acid-free tissue paper, put them in a box, and find a safe storage spot.

Don't trip over your past lives every morning to get to the present one!

A designer label isn't a valid reason for keeping clothes if you don't wear them. Yes, they cost a lot of money, but what purpose do they serve? Has the trend or novelty appeal vanished? The money you invested pays no dividends. Whisk each piece away *unless* it has possibilities as a vintage piece. Vintage designer clothes are all the rage and a niche market. Remember Julia Roberts picking up her Academy Award in a vintage Valentino gown, and Renée Zellweger in that gorgeous vintage gown at the Golden Globes? Look in the Yellow Pages under Vintage Clothes or check out eBay to see if you might get some money back.

"The future is now, bubbling with shining possibilities!"

Pay special attention to the condition of your "security blankets," those dependable outfits for tough days. Most of these favorites tend to be black or dark navy blue. One is your dress or pantsuit for days when you feel fat. Another is the no-brainer choice for days when you oversleep, are rushed and harried, or just plain can't get your brain in gear. These clothes are IMPORTANT to your psychic well-being, so be sure they are clean, pressed, fit, and ready to go—or head out tomorrow and find a replacement.

All right: now that you know what to look out for, let's begin!

THE ORGANIZATION BLUEPRINT

We know you may feel overwhelmed by what needs to be sorted, so take it one category at a time. Push back your clothes and clear a spot just for jackets. Then go from one end of the closet to the other, pulling out just the jackets. If you currently have them hanging with the skirt as a suit, separate them and hang each piece alone. A suit is one look, but jackets and skirts can match up with other pieces to create more options.

Next pull out all your pants and review them, followed by skirts, tops, sweaters and knits, then dresses. Separate and group each classification.

Dresses and casual tops need a critical eye. The fashion credibility of a dress gets dated quicker than any other piece because of style, detail, or length. Knit casual tops are often worn a lot and need frequent replacement. If you find a style you love, buy it in various colors and duplicate the basics such as black, white, or red.

Try things on in front of a full-length mirror. This is the only way you will know for sure what you want to do with each piece. Does it fit? Do you feel good wearing it? Are you happy with the fabric? Does it sag or dip? Inexpensive fabrics rarely age well. Fine, heavy fabrics such as cashmere aren't good choices if you've moved to the Sunbelt or have erratic hormones. If you've gained weight, can you ease the seams? If you have lost weight, you need alterations in fit and length.

Everyone gravitates toward a personal layout in her closet. You may wish to separate your work clothes from your casual and weekend wear: if so, then do it by classification. Either approach is more orderly when you arrange colors from light to dark. Skirts might be split into three groupings by length: mini, knee length, and longer. Split out bottoms into cropped pants and ankle length. Some women like to do tops by sleeve length. All your special occasion items can be grouped together at the far end of the closet or perhaps in another location.

Grab your handy notepad and keep a running "to do" list. By the end of this project you'll have clear directives about what needs to be repaired, what you need to buy, plus a shopping list of things you need to replace.

While your attention is focused on your closet, consider the simplest space-expanding step: double-hang half of it. Advertisements for closet companies show half of a closet filled with long items such as dresses and pants, while the other half has two bars: one above eye level and one below waist level, filled with short items such as tops, jackets, and skirts. Above these bars is usually a shelf. Separate this shelf into three sections: folded knits, handbags, and clear plastic storage boxes.

If you share your closet with a man, he'll also benefit by hanging jackets, shirts, and shorts on the double-hung section, and trousers and pants in the longer section. Organization and home improvement stores, as well as on-line companies offer easy-to-install system kits for closets.

Lighting is important in your closet. Good, bright overhead lighting

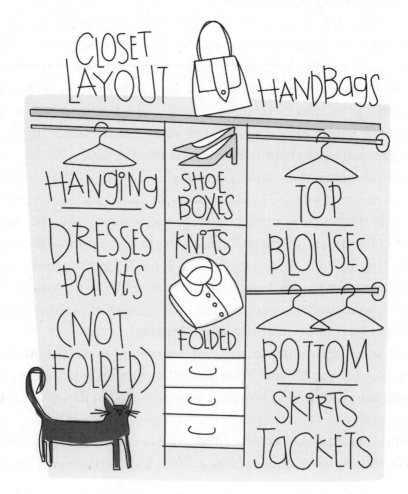

CLOSET LAYOUT HANDBAGS

HANGING
DRESSES
PANTS
(NOT
FOLDED)

SHOE BOXES
KNITS
FOLDED

TOP
BLOUSES
BOTTOM
SKIRTS
JACKETS

helps you discern shades of color. Doorjamb switches automatically turn lights on when a closet door opens. Track lighting outside a reach-in closet can be aimed toward specific sections.

Walk-in closets may be configured differently, based on size and the number of people sharing the closet. Besides dividing "his" and "her" hanging spaces into two sections each—one for long items and one with two bars—you may want to include smaller, vertically stacked storage slots for shoes or accessories. Check out vertical shoe storage bags with open fronts or vinyl windows. Hooks or Velcro straps wrap around closet rods, holding these nifty inventions in place. Built-in drawers are a storage boon and free up space in the bedroom. With enough space, you can also add built-in shoe bars at different levels, hanging storage squares or plastic boxes for folded knits, sweaters, and hats, and perhaps even a cedar-lined closed closet for out-of-season items.

ACCESSORIES ORGANIZATION

Accessories should be in plain view. If you don't see them, you forget what you own. Put shoes in clear plastic boxes on a shelf or stacked on the floor, arrange them on racks, in rows, or stowed in their original boxes with descriptive labels or a Polaroid picture glued on the end.

Arrange handbags vertically on your closet shelf, in view and in your consciousness. Buy cabinet storage organizers that you can stack on a shelf as a way to double space. Consider adding another shelf in your closet above the existing one.

Hang belts on circle rings or retractable horizontal belt racks with hooks. Similar racks may be utilized for long necklaces. It keeps them from getting tangled in your jewelry box. Just remember not to put belt and jewelry racks next to each other.

During your closet overhaul, make choices about where and how you want to store specific items. We advise placing tees, swimsuits, and exercise clothes in drawers. Sort items according to drawer size. One client with a nine-drawer lingerie chest sorts by athletic socks, trouser socks and panty hose, slips, bras, panties, tees, exercise bras, shorts and swimsuits, sweat suits, and knit pants. Sleepwear goes into the drawers in her bedside table.

Get your scarf collection out of a drawer. Maggie, a talented do-it-yourselfer, ties scarves around a vertical spring curtain rod placed at one end of her closet, from ceiling to floor. Evelyn, a superefficient manager, keeps favorite scarves looped around the blouses, jackets, or dresses she usually wears them with. Amy, an accessory collector, folds scarves and stacks them with her gloves and sunglasses in one of the hanging, windowed shoe-storage gizmos.

Laura, a pharmaceutical sales manager, fastened a grid on her swing-out closet door with a towel bar beneath it. Scarves go on the bar while necklaces hang from the grid alongside a long, three-inch-wide taffeta ribbon studded with her favorite blazer pins.

Jewelry storage is a challenge. Traditional multilevel jewelry boxes are never large enough and refuse to stay organized. We favor the convenience of larger shallow drawers with depths of two to three inches. Bedroom bureaus today often come with flat, velvet-lined drawers across the top, or you can create your own. A top drawer in a bedside table may work, or you could stack clear plastic trays with dividers. Plastic ice cube trays can double as containers for storing earrings or rings. Dividers protect your jewelry from scratching or damage.

Jewelry seems to have invisible tentacles attached to each woman's inner psyche. Admit it—you keep the oddest things in your jewelry boxes: foreign coins, unstrung pearls, odd stones, single earrings, garish bangle bracelets, wrong-size rings, watches with dead batteries, and hopelessly out-of-date earrings. Like your closet, this assortment is a microcosm of your life. On another day *after* you've cleaned out your closet, attack your jewelry collection. Once again, establish a nostalgia box (gifts from old boyfriends or inherited cameos, etc.), consignment items, broken pieces and dead watches, and a box of valuable items you don't wear often. The latter you take to a safety deposit box. You'll find more tips and hints about accessory storage and care in chapter 10, Punch Pieces and Finishing Touches.

You are not done yet! Immediately, right now—take your overflowing boxes and bags designated "Consignment" and "Charity" and put them in the car or by the front door. Do not hesitate. This step is an important part of the process and will prevent you from getting fainthearted and ruining what you have accomplished. No fair picking over the piles again!

A word of caution: check the pockets of each and every thing you send to consignment or charity. We've heard many sad tales. *Quinn tells of a visit from her brother who lives in San Francisco. He went to Disneyland overnight, and while he was gone she removed some cast-off clothes marked for charity donation from the guest room closet. The night he returned, her brother became distressed, demanding to know what happened to the clothes in the closet in*

"Shop in your own closet."

his room. Quinn told him she took them to the Salvation Army. "All my vacation money, three thousand dollars, was in the pocket of one jacket. I hid it there," he said. Fortunately, workers at the charity found the money and held it until Quinn arrived to pick it up the next day.

Vera, a traveling high-tech consultant, says she periodically checks her pockets, since she has a habit of stashing fifty to a hundred dollars in pockets of various suits when she travels, "So if someone steals my wallet or purse, I'll have cash."

Next, make an appointment with your seamstress for alterations, and drop off your laundry and dry cleaning on the same trip. You'll experience a wonderful sense of accomplishment. Plus, you'll have all these clean, fresh, fabulous-fitting outfits to wear!

THE PAYOFF!

The next two steps are fun, creative rewards for all your hard work. One, get on the phone and set up that swap party with your sisters or girlfriends. Remember how much fun you had in high school or college when you borrowed and swapped with one another and got great-looking outfits?

Step number two sounds funny if you've never tried it. Now that you have a clean, organized closet full of clothes that fit, we suggest you go shopping—in your closet. It is the most convenient and economical place to start. Get that notepad and pen and keep them handy. Chances are you ended up with a stash of things too good to pitch yet not quite right for your life today. For example, a corporate suit seems too stuffy for your new work-at-home consulting business. Most suit skirts and pants are basic in cut—could the skirt just happen to go with that new sweater set? Will a striped top zing up the pants? Could you wear the suit jacket with your jeans?

Look at each seemingly difficult piece with fresh eyes and a fresh perspective. Decide if it will go with something you already have, or if a single purchase will create a new outfit for you. Scan your color assortments and you'll be pleased to see how new combinations for outfits pop out. Take that beige and brown print top and hold it up to skirts or pants within the same color range. Exercise your hunches. Play with possibilities!

Another challenge is your accumulation of things that are in good shape but not quite *you* anymore. These represent expressions of a past fashion persona. Women evolve from season to season or year to year. You take up new hobbies such as making jewelry, hiking, or mountain biking. Some pastimes are messy and wreak havoc on clothing, others change your musculature, the fit of your clothes, or your concept of yourself. Your sister or friends may love your past persona items. Toss them in the swap box.

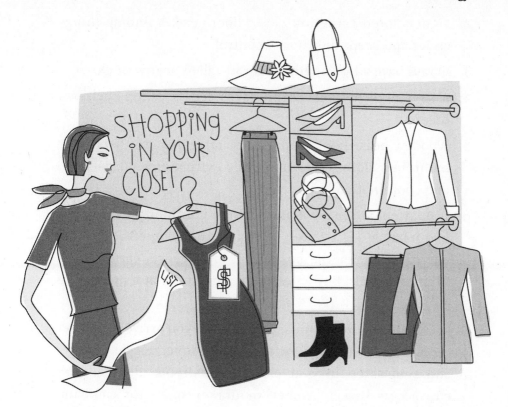

This fresh outlook can help you realize that perhaps a favorite outfit from last year looks a bit tired and needs to be moved from active duty to at-home work wear. If that's your decision, jot down a replacement on your list for a future shopping trip. There are reasons why you loved your old outfit enough to wear it so much. Figure out what they were and look for a replacement, not a whole new concept.

TIPS AND TRICKS FOR SETTING UP YOUR CLOSET

1. Keep a laundry pen handy to mark items on tags or inside shoes, belts or bags, to help you quickly discern black items from inky navy or brown. A simple *B, N,* or *BN* is a time-saver.

2. Light-colored carpet on closet floors makes finding things easier and keeps dust under control.

3. Always have a full-length mirror installed near your closet.

4. A step stool in your closet makes access to top shelves a breeze.

5. Wooden pegs, hooks, or a retractable bar are handy for bathrobes, clothes selection while getting dressed, packing, and coordination.

6. If quarters are really cramped then consider purchasing a bed frame at least eleven inches off the floor, creating storage space under the box spring for luggage, cartons, and other materials. Buy an extra long bed skirt at a linen store to conceal it.

7. Establish two drop points for use when you arrive home. Set up one near the door for keys, cell phone, pocket change, and sunglasses. In your closet or bedroom, designate an easy-access basket or shelf or drawer space for emptying your handbag, stashing your Palm Pilot, watch, eyeglasses, or contact case and other personal accessories.

8. Fold and stack your sweaters in categories such as sweater sets, by sleeve length, by neckline such as V neck or turtlenecks, and by heavyweight or cotton.

9. A simple chair or stool near the closet is handy for slipping on shoes and socks.

CHAPTER SIX

PROPORTION POLITICS: HORIZONTAL LINE DRESSING

Fashion is architecture: it is a matter of proportion.

COCO CHANEL, DESIGNER

The laments and self-sabotage that begin in front of the three-way mirror in clothing store dressing rooms all across the country sound the same.

"These pants are smiling at me. They're wayyy too tight."

"Yikes, this color looks awful on me!"

"I look like a blimp in this."

"Everything always hangs on me."

"I'm too old for this style. Don't they have anything for real women?"

"All I see are my boobs! But I liked the fabric on the rack."

"I'm too short for this. I look like I'm standing in a puddle."

"My fat neck makes me crazy."

"High water pants again. I'm *never* able to find pants long enough."

We rarely meet a woman who is happy with her body. Body image—not weight or age—is a woman's main concern. Almost every woman believes she is "hard to fit" in clothes because of a deficiency related to her proportions. It's the reason thousands of women hate to shop for clothes or become depressed with what they see in dressing room mirrors. Each one wishes to be taller, thinner, shorter, with longer legs, longer neck, bigger breasts, smaller breasts, narrower hips, lower waist—the list goes on.

These yearnings are debilitating to a woman's psyche.

When Judie was growing up in a small town on the Gulf Coast of

Florida, she loved to read Vogue *and* Harper's Bazaar. *Each opened a window to a magical world of fashion and sophistication. "At the age of twelve and thirteen, I was really funny, skinny, and gawky-looking. Diana Vreeland, then editor of* Vogue, *issued one of her famous fashion decrees: "Long necks. This season it is long necks." I looked at pictures of Audrey Hepburn, and then looked in the mirror in despair. For weeks I walked around doing neck exercises—chin up—stretching, stretching—trying to achieve the impossible. And when I didn't succeed, I felt doomed to be forever an ugly duckling.*

Women convince themselves that losing ten or twenty pounds would make a difference. But even if you lose weight, you will still be the same height, your legs will still be short or long, your waist will stay in the same place, and your shoulders will be either narrow or broad.

Losing weight, gaining weight, lifting weights, and liposuction will not change the length of your legs, the position of your waist, the arch of your neck, or the width of your hip-

Women always think something is wrong with them. They never think something is wrong with the clothes.

bones. Like eye color and curly or straight hair, your body proportions are predetermined. Your ancestry determines your skeletal structure; you are your mother and father, grandmothers and grandfathers. Body proportions are insidious, because "shortcomings" created by proportions can seem to be personal faults.

Jackie was out of college and into her career before she discovered something important about herself. While a couture buyer, she had occasion to work with a colleague named Kay Clifford. Jackie envied Kay's appearance in clothes. They seemed to hang on her just like a model's. Jackie's clothes did not, despite the fact both she and Kay were five feet eight and a half inches tall, wore the same size, and weighed exactly the same. One day she summoned up the nerve to ask Kay how she always managed to look picture perfect. Kay stood up from her desk, walked out on the floor to a full-length mirror, and said, "Stand by me. Now, see the difference? You are short-waisted and I am long-waisted." Jackie looked and immediately realized her waistline was about three inches higher on her torso than Kay's natural waistline. It was all about proportion.

Think about how off-the-rack clothes fit you. Are sleeves always too long? Pant legs never long enough? Do blouses not stay tucked in? Turtlenecks strangle? Do waistlines on jackets and dresses never hit where they are supposed to fit? Hemlines droop, making you look like you are standing in a hole? Swimsuits slip up, up, up, despite constant tugs down? Pleated Bermuda shorts fit like they begin under your bust? Do clothes seem skimpy in length or bunch up around your waist?

The fact is your body proportions may be making you feel uncomfortable in your clothes. But that's fixable.

At the age of thirteen, Cynthia sprouted up to her full height of five feet eight inches. Buying jeans or pants long enough was a struggle. She always felt uncomfortable and habitually tugged on her pant legs, trying to make them longer. Every mirrored surface gave her a chance to see if her ankles were sticking out. As an adult, Cynthia's search for pants with extra long legs was a constant challenge. When capri pants became trendy, Cynthia couldn't bear trying them on, as the short length brought back painful childhood memories. Judie presented a solution— order pants in tall sizes. Correctly, Cynthia had never classified herself as a "tall" size, yet with her long legs and inseam measurement (inseam length is determined by measuring from the crotch seam to the bottom of pants) she is a "tall" size in pants.

The key in dealing with body proportions is learning what looks best on you, making sure your clothes fit correctly, and knowing how to find what you need. Once you know your proportions, shopping and dressing become easier. Never compromise the proportions that work for you, despite fashion trends.

*I write about clothes as magical
things that can change you.*

JUDITH KRANTZ, AUTHOR

So, it's time to break out the magic wand called Horizontal Line Dressing. By experimenting with clothing, you will learn how to create visual illusions on your body so that you feel good in your clothes and look your best. It really works!

Patty Sturgis, a highly successful business owner, decided to run for public office. She called Jackie in for consultations. After three meetings, a closet gutting, and several shopping trips, the compliments came rolling in. "It was remarkable," said Patty. "Everyone would look at me strangely but in a most flattering way and say things like 'You've lost weight,' or 'What have you done to yourself?' I hadn't lost a pound, unfortunately, but I had followed the Horizontal Line Dressing formula to the letter. It transformed my appearance."

Gather round and learn how you can transform yourself.

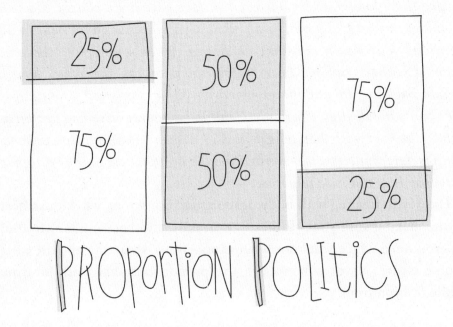

PROPORTION POLITICS

COMFORT BOXES AND WHAT THEY MEAN TO YOU

This simple balancing act is all about skillfully layering the horizontal lines of your clothing on your body.

Imagine your body from the top of your shoulders to the floor, closely surrounded by the lines of a tall, vertical rectangle. Visualize the rectangle empty. We're going to look at the space from your shoulders to your waist and your waist to the floor, drawing a horizontal line across the box at your waist.

Dressed in your bra and panties, exercise gear, or a leotard, stand in front of a full-length mirror. Is the longest space from your waist to the floor? If so, you are a 25/75-body type. A 50/50-body type is a fairly evenly divided body frame with 50 percent of the body above the waist, 50 percent below. If you have long body length, a low waist and shorter legs, you are a 75/25-body type.

Can't decide? Try this. Place your arms at your sides with palms facing backward. Raise your arms, keeping your elbows pressed in at your sides. Look or feel where your waist falls in relation to your elbow. If your waist is above your elbow, you are short-waisted. If it falls exactly at your elbow then you are conventional-waisted, and if it is below your elbow you have a long waist.

Jackie was speaking about body proportion at a women's conference and asked for a volunteer to come up and be measured. Rosalind came forward. Jackie determined that the woman was long-waisted, and then explained what style jackets are best for this figure type. Suddenly Rosalind interrupted and said in an emotional voice, "Excuse me, but my mother always said I was short-waisted and I believed it. All my life I've had difficulty finding clothing, because apparently I was looking for the wrong proportions."

A year later Jackie did a return engagement in the same city, and again the topic was proportion. "Some women are not familiar with their true proportions and make their bodies appear to be different than what they are," she said, and related the story of Rosalind. A woman in the back of the room stood up and said, "I am that woman." The beautifully dressed woman was totally transformed. She stood tall and walked to the stage with an air of confidence. "After you changed my perception of myself last year," said Rosalind, "I saw myself in a new way; and suddenly everything changed."

Are you still uncertain about your proportions? Measure the distance between your bottom rib and the top of your hipbone. If the distance is one or two inches you are short-waisted and thus a 25/75-body type. An approximate two- to three-inch difference indicates you are a 50/50-body type. If the distance is four or five inches you are long-waisted and a 75/25-body type.

Look at our diagram examples. If you are long-waisted, you have more space to deal with on your upper body. If you are short-waisted, you have less. More available space enables you to use larger items and put in more detail. In smaller spaces, you must reduce the size of items and/or use less or smaller detail. A 75/25 woman can wear more on her upper body and pile on accessories, while a 25/75 must be acutely conscious of avoiding too much detail, using smaller-scale accessories, and fewer of them. Of course, the reverse is also true. A 25/75 has long legs and more space to play with on her lower body. A 50/50 woman is less concerned with proportion issues, but we rarely meet such fortunate women.

We call our diagrams Comfort Boxes because each category has things those women are comfortable wearing and things that are uncomfortable for them to wear. So let's begin to find what's perfect for you!

A 25/75 has longer legs than other body types, and this leg length creates an illusion of being taller. Hooray! But your shorter torso causes tops and blouses to bunch up around your waist and under your bust. You feel chubby and constricted. Sizable collars swallow you up, and wide belts are instruments of torture. Jackets off the rack never hit body contours correctly. Shaped waists drop near hipbones, enlarging your silhouette into a shapeless blob. Fitted dresses crumple with excess fabric at the waist, and their stitched-in darts go up and over your bust. Many women with short waists are so frustrated by this that they give up on wearing dresses. A woman with a short waist and large bust is even more miserable, as her midriff and waist vanish under fabric falling over her ample breasts. A goal for a 25/75 is to visually lengthen the upper torso, bringing the body in balance.

We suggest that 25/75 women scout around a favorite store and seek out the petite or petite plus departments. These designations are based on proportion, *not* on height. Both classifications are cut to fit women with short waists. Jackets, tops, and blouses run shorter in length and may fit you perfectly. Again, this is an exploration project. Try on several different manufacturers and go up and down in size. We find this works best on short-sleeve or sleeveless tops. Jackets are problematical, as long sleeves also run shorter, but you may get lucky.

A 75/25 is long-waisted and easier to fit. Your challenge is blouses, jackets, vests, and swimsuits being too short. Things constantly pull and will not stay tucked in. Short jackets and vests stop inches above the waist, making them look too small or skimpy on your body. Cropped fitted blouses bare skin at the waist. Small breasts coupled with a low waistline make a 75/25 feel less shapely and more flat chested. Wide belts, inset and shaped waistbands, and detail on the upper torso from below the bust to the shoulder are all good ways to raise your waistline and crop your upper body length.

Leg length for a 75/25 is short, making it important to avoid anything cutting across the leg, such as pedal pushers, capris, ankle and midcalf boots, ankle or T-strap shoes. The sleekest, simplest line from waist to floor will make your legs look longer. When pants puddle on the floor because they are too long, have them tailored, without cuffs, to fall over your higher heeled shoes, and wear trouser socks that are the same color as your pants. As an experiment try petite size pants, which are cut shorter, or look for pants designated as short.

A 50/50 body type generally has fewer concerns unless her waist and/or bust are not well defined, creating a straight up-and-down silhouette. The challenge there is to create curves or waist definition.

MOVING THE LINES TO CREATE YOUR MOST FLATTERING VISUAL IMPRESSION

Six horizontal lines are key to the visual illusion of Horizontal Line Dressing: the neck/shoulder, waist, wrist, skirt hem, pant length, and jacket length. Paying attention to each line is imperative to visually making you look your best. Learning to balance the top half of your body in relation to the bottom half is key to achieving the most pleasing vertical line, making you look taller and evenly proportioned. Think of it as asset management—making the most of what you have.

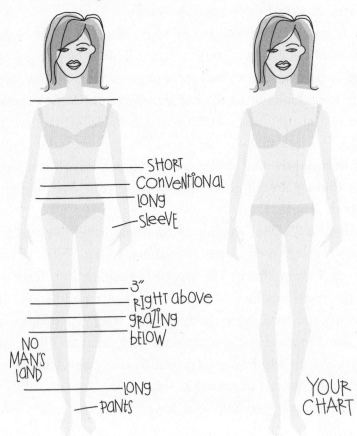

SHORT
CONVENTIONAL
LONG
SLEEVE

3"
RIGHT above
GRAZING
bELOW

NO MAN'S LAND

LONG
PANTS

YOUR CHART

1. The Neck and Shoulder

Your Neck

This space is our first focus, as your neckline is a framing device for your upper torso. Look at your neck space, from under your chin to your clavi-cle bones. Is the space limited or long? Is there enough space so you feel comfortable wearing turtlenecks or choker necklaces? If not, you can learn tricks to elon-gate this space, like lowering the lines of your neckline to show more skin.

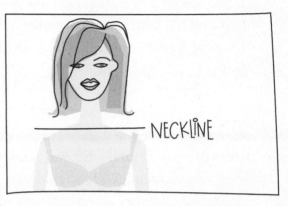

The amount of skin you expose not only attracts attention, but also diverts it. For example, bare shoulders or a top exposing one shoulder rivets attention, while a bare back stops the eye from noticing much else. At your neckline, the amount of skin you reveal and the style of collars you wear can make a dramatic difference in balancing your body propor-tions. High band collars and turtlenecks are almost universally flattering. Both styles are a perfect frame for most faces. A slim V neck makes the neck appear longer and is equally flattering. A collar flipped up in back adds a few inches to the length of the torso. V necks, scoop-neck tops, and unbuttoned, open collars visually lengthen your neckline. Softly draped shell blouses or the crisscross of a wrap or draped blouse is a sophisti-cated way to achieve the same effect. In warmer weather, sundresses with straps, tube, and tank tops open up your neck space. Layering camisoles or tank tops under open shirts, or shirts knotted or buttoned just above the waist, also trick the eye. Long necklaces, pendant drops, and twenty-six-inch-length pearls similarly lengthen the appearance of your neck space.

If you never felt your neck was long or short, you probably are conventional and have learned by trying (or should) what works best for you.

For centuries romantic literature praised women with long necks, deeming them elegance and grace personified. If you have a long neck, draw attention to it with beautiful earrings and necklaces, scarves, rolled collars, turtlenecks, cowl necks, and shoulder-baring evening looks. Wide antique-style collar necklaces, lacy-banded collars, and upswept hairstyles subtly allude to the romantic allure of this swanlike feature.

Shoulder Width

Shoulder width is a significant horizontal line. Women born with broad shoulders are naturally blessed, while others acquire them through sports such as swimming. Wide shoulders are a body bonus, as clothes hang or drape from them as designers intended.

Think of an inverted triangle with the V-point at your feet. This is the configuration you want to achieve when placing horizontal lines against your body. The widest visual point should be across your shoulder line, narrowing down at the lower leg and shoes. Width—actual or visual width—at your shoulder line makes your waist and hips appear smaller.

Shoulder pads are the best way for women with narrow or sloping shoulders to even out dimensions. If this is your body type, shoulder pads are always "in style." Do not go to the extreme of football pads. Experiment with several sizes and styles of shoulder enhancers, such as rounded and squared pads. Try them on with different items in your wardrobe until you hit the magic ones doing the most to equalize your dimensions. Generally more rounded shapes work with knits and soft fabrics, while tailored shirts and jackets look best with square-edge shoulder pads. We know women who swear by camisoles or bras sold with attached shoulder pads. When buying a new top, never assume the shoulder pads sewn in are the right shoulder pads for you. Try it on, scrutinize the shape in the mirror, and if they don't work, snip them out and wear your own pads. You'll find an array of different styles in the notions department of most fabric stores.

Emily, a friend of ours who is a model, is addicted to the magic of shoulder pads. She says they do so much for her silhouette—and self-confidence—that she puts them in all her clothes, including bathrobes.

Horizontal stripes on sweaters and knit tops are also effective ways to create visual balance. Try a single horizontal stripe or several stripes across your shoulders and bust line to counterbalance wider hips. Boat neck tops, deep V necks, or wide scooped-neck tees maximize your shoulders while minimizing the waist and hips. Short or cap sleeves extend the perception of wider shoulders.

Halter-style tops emphasize vertical lines while revealing skin, creating the effect of broader shoulder space. Asymmetrical cuts such as one-shoulder tops lengthen the horizontal shoulder line across one shoulder to the lower neck, then down the chest and under the arm.

Artfully cut stripes in diagonal patterns ripple and confuse the eye into believing shoulder space is wider. Bold color blocks or argyle patterns enhance the perceived size of your upper torso too.

2. The Waist Line

Historically, beautiful women possessed tiny waists—remember Scarlett O'Hara? Today women eschew corsets, and a natural shape reigns. Still, women envy those lucky beauties with diminutive waists. It's fine to be

proud of your small waistline, and if you have one, dress to show it off—but carefully. The location of your waist impacts your appearance far more than its circumference. Regardless of height, a small waistline makes ample hips or bustline

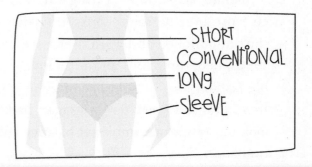

appear bigger. If you are five feet tall, emphasizing a small waistline draws everyone's eyes down and underscores your shortness and tiny stature.

If you have a long waist, your goal is to shorten the appearance of your torso by wearing wide waistbands, belts, and layering in—which means wearing the longest item closest to your body and adding shorter items over it. The top layer could be a bolero or wispy vest. Lifted waistlines or slight empire styles on dresses and tops flatter you and create the desired illusion. At the same time, you want to visually lengthen your lower body by wearing long slim skirts, narrow pants, and higher heels.

If you have a short waist, most likely you have long legs. Smile, because women with other type figures would kill to have your leg proportion! The trick is to make your upper body visually stretch to balance your lower body length.

The easiest way to do this is to use tops that seem to add a couple of extra inches in length. Most women have a specific way they like to wear their tops, or they wear them that certain way through force of habit. Generally there are two types: the tuckers and the nontuckers. *"I always tuck my tops in. If I don't I feel sloppy," said a woman in Kansas. "Well, actually, now that I think about it, my mom always told me and my brother to tuck that shirttail in."*

If you want to tuck your blouse or top in and still lengthen your look, try the blouson trick. Blouson means to ease out a little bit of tucked-in fabric so it falls over the belt line, extending the color, print, or texture of the top. This works wonders on men too.

Nontuckers utilize layering out. It is similar camouflage to open jackets worn over narrower tops with skirts or pants skimming the body. A shirt unbuttoned and worn over a tee blurs body definition. In the early 1990s, long tunic tops and extra long sweaters over slim pants became a big fashion look. It sold like crazy as the fashion industry rolled with a trend that hid every flaw a woman had. Actually, this *long over narrow* look illustrates one universal balance rule, closely akin to another: *long over short.*

Women with short waists appear more balanced in tops that fall an inch or two below the waist or to the hipbone. They can skim, but not hug, the body. You may need to have shell tops or vests altered and shortened to find your most flattering length. Skirts and tops without waistbands, the kind tailored to fit just below the waist, are a smart choice for this figure type. Those in great shape may experiment with short-rise-pant styles.

3. The Wrist

Sleeve length can make or break the impression a woman conveys. Costume designers use sleeves as a device to manipulate character impression. Make them slightly too short and you look a bit bumpkinlike, with protruding wrist bones and poorly fitting clothing. Make sleeves long and sloppy and one looks clownish, or like a street urchin adrift in a grown man's clothes. These are not impressions that a well-dressed woman wishes to convey.

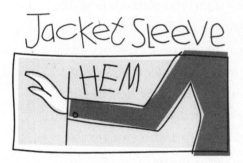

We believe in narrower sleeves on jackets and tops, because long, narrow sleeves create strong vertical lines from your shoulders to your hips, creating an optical illusion of elongating the body. Narrow sleeves break the upper body into three parts by providing "see through" between the sleeves and the body of the jacket or blouse, and both techniques contribute to making you appear taller and slimmer.

Finding your perfect sleeve length is easy. Place your arms at your sides with palms facing backward. Keeping your arms and elbows fairly close to your body, bend your arms at the elbows until your forearms are perpendicular to the floor and your hands straight out, with palms facing down. Now bend your hands upward at the wrist, as if you are about to push something away. The line of your long sleeves should fall exactly at the crease at the wrist.

To achieve this precise line in tailored clothing may require alterations, shortening or lengthening sleeves. Shirts can be modified to hit on the right line by simply moving the button or buttons to make them tighter around the wrist. You may want blouses with fuller, or too long, sleeves tapered by a seamstress for a slimmer look. Deep, narrow cuffs or fitted sleeves make the arm appear slimmer.

With the proper neckline, three-quarter-length or long sleeves provide good figure balance for women who carry more body weight below their waist than above.

If your wrists and forearms are small, then revealing skin space at the wrist in blouses, tops, and sweaters with long sleeves is effective in creating optical illusions. Simply push up or roll up the sleeves and let the taper of your arms and wrists help you look slimmer.

During spring and summer you may opt for a variety of sleeve lengths. Just where you place your sleeve depends on how shapely and toned your arms appear. Most women make their decision based on a comfort level. Many of our clients and midlife women ask: *Should I go sleeveless or not?* A considerable number spend hours working out in gyms or health clubs just so they can show off their arms. One aerobics instructor explained the logic. "If you have good-looking shoulders and arms, you can get away with a lot more that's wrong someplace else on your body."

In southern Sunbelt states, simmering climates dictate the necessity of less fabric or sleeve much of the year. Do you opt for comfort in heat or cover-up? The choice is yours. Jackie always asks women what they think about sleeve length as well as all their proportions. And she finds the individual always has the answer.

Fashion trends move sleeve lengths up and down, but long sleeves are classic, and knowing your correct personal horizontal wrist line is valuable information for looking your best.

4. The Skirt Hemline

Skirt lengths generate more fashion and appearance controversy than any other single dimension in women's clothing. Minis, maxis, weekend wear, corporate dressing, designer dictates, and appropriateness—even the world of sports gets into the act. Today there are no hard-and-fast rules. Yet there are still guidelines.

For business and community activities, hemlines raise eyebrows if the horizontal line is more than three inches above the knee. Anything shorter is short for a reason: to be eye-catching, sexy, flirty, sporty, or perfect for a game of tennis.

A hem that hits at the knee or grazes the knee is versatile, as various jacket lengths look good with this classic length. To be specific, this length covers half of the knee and leaves half of the knee showing. If you are not happy with your knees, drop the graze to just below the knee.

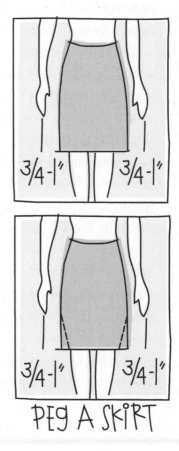

PEG A SKIRT

For women with great-looking legs, these just-grazing-the-knee or slightly above-the-knee skirts become interesting if they have off-center, side, or back slits. A caution: skirts with front slits have a way of embarrassing every woman who ever wears them.

We customarily suggest our clients "peg" their straight skirts. This is a subtle, effective alteration. Before getting your skirt altered, make a quick check to see if the skirt is already pegged. Hold it up by each side of the waistline, straight in front of you, and notice if it seems to get narrower toward the hemline. If it goes in there, it is already pegged. If not, try it on and drop your hands at your sides with palms facing your thigh. From the tip of your middle finger to the hemline, take the side seams in one-quarter to one-half inch. To instantly see how this trick works, stand in front of a full-length mirror in a straight skirt and reach back and pull the lower part of your skirt back. Shazam! You appear taller and thinner. In magazines and catalogs, models always have their skirts pulled back and clipped with clothespins or clips, because it creates a more flattering line and makes the clothes look better.

We'll admit it. We are not fond of midcalf lengths. Midcalf-length skirts only work if they are fanciful, such as tiered western prairie or beach 'n' sandals styles, bias-cut, fluid long skirts inspired by movies such as *Out of Africa* or vintage-tinged tea dresses. Prairie skirts and long, bias looks come off best when worn with boots. Sarong-style beach looks and handkerchief hems demand open-sandal-style shoes or heels. Tea dresses need a demure ballet slipper or Mary Jane–style pump.

Straight midcalf-length skirts are deadly and unflattering. The horizontal hemline hits at the fattest part of the lower leg, tending to add years and weight to one's overall silhouette and appearance. Watch a woman walking down the street in a straight, tailored, midcalf-length skirt. She looks like she is wearing a tent with two animals fighting inside.

Ankle-length skirts have more drawbacks than pluses. While they do extend the body silhouette to its longest length, it is tough to whip through a busy day—especially in an urban environment—in an ankle-grabbing piece of fabric. Long skirts are best for casual wear, at-home dinner parties, or poolside. Many women feel comfortable in a long skirt because they avoid showing their knees, calves, or ankles. Ankle-length sarong-style and wrap skirts are good picks for visual tomfoolery. The eye perceives the steep, diagonal line formed by the sarong as near vertical, and thus slimming and lengthening. Wrap styles with vertical bands or print designs break the lower body into two parts while elongating the line from waist to ankle. Femme fatales like long skirts with slits up the side to midthigh.

A long, plain straight skirt turns your body silhouette into a blocky rectangle. Study your reflection in a full-length mirror and then decide for yourself.

5. Pant Length

Fact: Today in the United States, 90 percent of all women wear trousers 50 percent of the time. That means when women reach into their closets for a daily dose of self-esteem, they gravitate to the comfort, versatility, and ease of pants. So pay heed and learn the best way for *you* to wear pants.

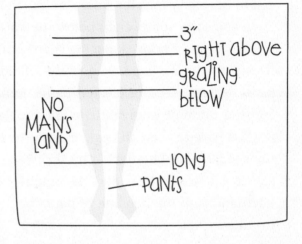

To achieve your most flattering line, the hemline of full-length pants or trousers should fall in front to the top of the shoe or break slightly at the shoe, allowing the back to fall approximately at the midpoint of the back of the shoe. Occasionally we see pants tailored slightly longer in the back, down the heel. Shorter women especially like this trick with higher heels, as the lift gives added stature. This, again, is a personal choice. We do not encourage it for all women because the longer material is subject to more wear and tear from shoes, curbs, and inclement weather.

To create the longest, leanest silhouette, stockings or trouser socks and shoes should be the same color as the pants. Always determine the length of pants by wearing the shoes you intend to wear with those pants.

Whether to cuff or not is a personal decision. Cuffs do cut the elongated line you may be after. Generally cuffs look best on pants that are a bit narrower at the bottom, allowing the pants to drape elegantly over the shoe. Narrow-leg pants taper the bottom of your silhouette, giving you that desired inverted triangle and making you look taller and slimmer.

Petite women, five feet four inches and under, can enhance their height by wearing narrow-leg pants and avoiding cuffs. Wide pant legs, because of their blocky shape, look best on taller women, as their height balances the proportion.

You must pick and choose among a smorgasbord of choices, as the definition of "fashion pants" fluctuates each season, with pant legs constantly growing narrower or flared, boot cut, or shorter, inching up the calf to become capri, toreadors, or gauchos.

If you carry your weight below the waistline, opt for trouser pants with soft pleats and a body-skimming shape or flat-front pants with an eased fit. If your thighs are large, your body will appear more balanced in pleated pants. When selecting pleated pants, look for a malleable rayon or wool crepe or ultrafine wool fabric to fall into flattering vertical drape lines.

You have to keep an eagle eye on the length of pants and trousers, as their length can be affected by shrinkage if you wash them and by weight fluctuations. If the hemline of pants or trousers is tailored to fall at the instep and you gain or lose weight, you'll notice the length of your pants rise or fall accordingly.

In chapter 7, Building a Wardrobe from the Bottoms Up, we examine in greater detail the ins and outs of selecting the right style pant or trouser for different figure types.

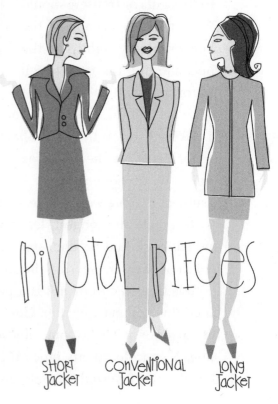

PIVOTAL PIECES

SHORT Jacket   CONVENTIONAL Jacket   LONG Jacket

6. Jacket Length and Shape

We call the jacket the pivotal piece, because a jacket is the ultimate finishing touch for an outfit and usually the single most expensive item in a woman's wardrobe. Women collect jackets for a variety of reasons. They get cold. They need this piece for a business dress code requirement. Jackets also hide a variety of imagined body flaws, thus making a woman feel more secure. Yet many women do not know how to wear a jacket or select one that will flatter them the most. It is all in the way you layer the proportions and horizontal line of a jacket against your body structure. You can bring out the magic of a properly proportioned jacket by studying several points.

Length

Stand in front of a full-length mirror wearing a tee top and slim-fitting pants. Place your arms at your sides, palms inward. Make a fist, then slide your arms around to the back of your body, and turn almost backward to the mirror. You should find that the knuckle line is exactly at the position your leg begins. This is the length you want to wear the horizontal hemline of your jacket for maximum flattery. It is the length that plays up your entire leg length while covering what you are less comfortable revealing. *This line is especially important if you carry more weight below your waistline.*

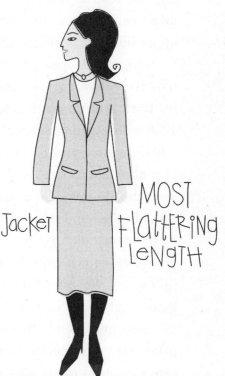

You do not want to wear a jacket longer than this because the lower hemline cuts your leg length, making you appear shorter and wider. This is a key line for most petite size women. The only exception would be a short-waisted petite, meaning you have a short waistline and longer legs. Then you may inch your jacket slightly downward.

Petites with even, 50/50 proportions may choose to wear shorter jackets in different styles. It's a good practice to always look at yourself in a three-way mirror to see where the hemline of the jacket lays across the back.

As a woman's height and leg length increases, so may the length of her jacket. Every three years or so, fashion trends dabble with midthigh- or midcalf-length jackets, sweaters, or sleeveless vests. Keep your personal proportion policies firmly in mind when trying on these varying lengths.

Fit

The most flattering fit for a jacket is skimming the body. Most women need some alteration by a good tailor to achieve this look. Keep in mind, proper fit will make your jacket look more expensive and you will feel better in your clothes.

A classic soft blazer style with narrow shawl lapels, single button closing, and seminarrow sleeves creates flattering lines: a deep V in front and diagonal lines from the armpit to the hem of the jacket, breaking up the upper body. A collarless jacket with V front creates similar lines.

A high envelope-style neckline or mandarin collar jacket slims the silhouette with its narrow shape and body-contoured seams midfront and in the back. If buttons are hidden under a placket in front, the placket forms a flattering, strong vertical line down the middle of the jacket. A row of striking buttons forms a bolder vertical line.

Short jackets are best on slim-hipped women. If you want to try to wear short jackets, be cautious. Keep tailoring or detail focused on your shoulder line and upper body. The lower part of the jacket and hem must be the same color as the skirt or pant. This keeps the eye from seeing the break between the top and bottom and perceives them as one continuous silhouette. We especially like shorter jackets worn in monochromatic tones, such as a creamy yellow jacket and pants worn with a burnt golden silk shantung shell blouse, or a brown short jacket and pants worn over a beige knit top. Mixing textures is sophisticated and tantalizes the eye. One exception to matching the jacket to your pants would be when you dress to the inside, by wearing a top in the same color as the pants. In this case, your jacket may contrast in color or texture.

Your bustline is an important factor in proper jacket fit. Ideally the tips of your breasts should appear to be roughly an equal distance from the top of your shoulders to your waistline. Often the easiest way to accomplish an adjustment is through shortening or lengthening your bra shoulder straps. That's one reason why bra straps adjust. You don't just put them in place once and wear them that way until you pitch the bra.

Wearing the proper style bra is essential, as jackets tend to look a little weird if you put a décolleté push-up bra under a conservative blazer. Generally a bra with a seamless molded cup or a smooth cup lace model is best under jackets.

Body shapers can lift, shape, separate, and flatten, but even Lycra and spandex have limits. Minimize your bust with bras designed to minimize, bras cleverly designed and seamed to hold and suppress. Most guarantee to make you look one cup size smaller.

Breasts change as you move through life. Their size is sometimes influenced by medications such as birth control pills or estrogen supplements, or by physical changes such as having children, weight gain and weight loss, as well as the natural aging process.

Be certain your jacket easily closes or buttons over your bust. A top that pulls and strains at buttonholes or gapes open kills any look.

Many large-busted women choose to wear soft, unconstructed jackets because this type of jacket flatters their body proportions by falling smoothly and gracefully from the shoulder over their upper body. Other women like the style for reasons of climate or personal comfort. Often these soft jackets are less expensive and offer a fresh alternative look to your wardrobe. The term "unconstructed" means a softer shoulder line, looser silhouette, and a more casual appearance while still creating a finished outfit. In general, unconstructed jackets are minimally lined or not lined at all. Unconstructed jackets in knits, cotton, or rayon weaves, and bright prints come off as sporty or less formal than such jackets made of linen, silk, satin, or wool crepe.

Every few fashion cycles, cardigan sweaters emerge as a viable alternative to jackets. They appear as matching pieces to a tank, short-sleeved, or V-necked sweater in a twin set, or they stand alone in bulkier knits as a jacket substitute. Cardigans of varying length, from hipbone, midthigh, or midcalf, tend not to supply body coverage, because of a sweater's innate body consciousness.

Big and oversize shirts worn over tee tops or camisoles as layering pieces provide extra polish for casual outfits and coverage for the wearer, making them feel more confident. In choosing such lightweight alternatives to a jacket, keep your horizontal lines in mind.

Now, a Quick Exercise!

Go to your closet and pull out your favorite jacket, blouse, knit top, pants, skirt, and dress. Pick up each piece and ask yourself these questions: Why is this my favorite piece? How does this item make me *feel* when I wear it?

There is an extremely important emotional reason why you consider each item your favorite. Each item may make you feel confident, slimmer, taller, prettier, comfortable, or flattered.

Gwynn told us this story: one morning as she was getting dressed for work, she was pulling clothes out of her closet and tossing them on the bed as she looked for her "good pants." Her husband, Steve, looked on quizzically, then said, "You've got fifteen pairs of black pants. Just pick one." "But I knew I needed this one particular pair of pants today," recounted Gwynn. "Steve thought I was crazy."

We would bet money you see yourself in that story. You own five pairs of black pants or blue jeans, but want one particular pair on a certain day for a certain reason.

Judie owns seven sweatshirts, yet on a recent cold morning she sorted through them all until she found the big, baggy black one with the ragged neck. "I was going to be writing at home all day and it makes me *feel* comfortable," was her reason.

Look again at each of your favorite pieces until you figure out why it earns that distinction. The neckline may be the most flattering. The color sets off your coloring. The jacket fits you just right. The skirt is exactly the perfect length for your leg. The pants are a great fabric and drape just right for your proportions. The dress always makes you feel sharp. Now that you realize what each item does for you, go back to our tips on horizontal lines. You'll discover you already knew some of the points outlined. You *feel* which lines look best on you.

SAY YES, SAY NO

YES — SHORT NECK?	NO
Unbuttoned collars	Turtleneck
Slim V neck	Cowl neck
Scoop neck	Scarf tied at neck

YES — NARROW SHOULDERS?	NO
Shoulder pads	Vertical stripes
Boat necks	Jumper
Wide V neck	Form-fitting tops
Short and cap sleeves	Halter tops

YES — LARGE BUST?	NO
Contour jacket with vertical seams	Bold prints on top
Dress with long sleeve	Long necklaces
Well-fitting bra	Shiny fabrics on top

YES — SMALL BUST?	NO
Pockets at bustline	Form-fitting clothing
Detail on tops	Bustier or strapless
Bust-enhancing bras	Deep necklines

YES	SHORT WAIST?	NO
Long top over bottom		Tucking tops tightly
Blouson blouses or shirts		Wide belts
Remove belt loops		Short fitted jackets

YES	LONG WAIST?	NO
Wide belt		Belt that matches top
Jacket to hipbone		Short jackets
Tall sizes		Brief miniskirts

YES	NO WAIST?	NO
No waistbands		Midriff tops
Blouson at waist		Tucking tops tightly
Third piece to camouflage		Belts with two-piece outfit

YES	5'4" OR SHORTER?	NO
Dress in one color		Three-quarter-length jackets
Dress to inside		Flat shoes with long skirt
Vertical stripe		A-line or full skirts

YES	PEAR SHAPED?	NO
Dark bottoms		Light-color bottoms
Diagonal stripes		Large prints on bottom
Shoulder pads		Tight-fitting bottoms
Three-quarter or long sleeves		Pleated skirts

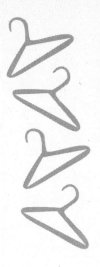

CHAPTER SEVEN

BUILDING A WARDROBE FROM THE BOTTOMS UP

A beautiful woman is someone who pays a lot of attention to herself and knows what suits her.

VIVIAN WESTWOOD, BRITISH DESIGNER

Early in my personal shopping business, I learned that the bottom is the hardest place to fit," says Jackie. *"It was really driven home for me when one of my first clients booked me for several hours of consultation with her sister, a New Yorker planning a move to Florida. In advance, and armed with my client's sizes, I gathered up a variety of pieces that could ease Sarah into her new Florida casual lifestyle. Her "try on" session started in the dressing room of a favorite department store.*

We started with the tops—all of them worked! Everyone was thrilled—until we got to the bottoms. Here, NOTHING seemed to work. Sarah bemoaned the alternately tight, baggy, and otherwise ill fit of every bottom she tried on. Frustration mounted for Sarah, her sister, and myself as she tried on eight different pants and walk shorts.

Finally: "Let's start over," I said. I located a variety of styles of trousers, skirts, and shorts, and we didn't stop until we had the perfect fit for Sarah's body. Unfortunately, this meant we had to start all over again for tops. THAT was my moment of realization. From that day forward, I always start at the bottom and build a wardrobe upward.

Most shopping trips begin with a familiar scenario. You set out with a fantasy in your mind's eye: beautiful new outfits for a new season. You gather up things to try on and go into a fitting room. It's drab and gloomy, the only light emanates from a flickering fluorescent tube. Faded green

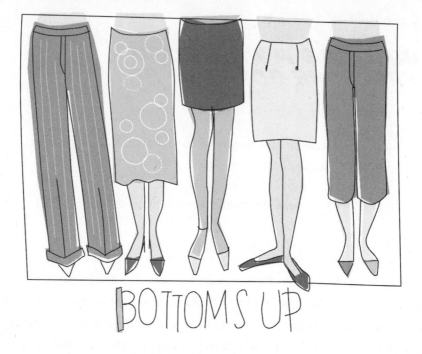

walls and the frayed carpet smell of chalk and dust. One hook is broken. Only one person can fit in the narrow space behind the banging shutter door. The cubicle is so cramped, the mirror invades your personal space. Each day, dressing rooms such as these breed epidemics of depression, anxiety attacks, and delusional body-image perceptions. Such plagues peak during swimsuit season.

You start by trying on bottoms. The first pants are tight at the hips, the second strain at the waistband, and the jeans are impossible to zip up. Your image in the mirror bulges, self-confidence deflates. Smack down—no wish fulfillment.

Your reaction is predictable. "I've gained weight." "I'm bloated." "I shouldn't have eaten that (dinner) (cake) (ice cream) last night." "I'm going to seed; I've got middle-age spread." "I've got to get back on a diet." You slink out of the store in a funk—dismayed, dejected, depressed.

The funny thing is, you *don't* get devastated when the *top* is too tight. Bigger breasts are good. Watch yourself and your friends as you try on clothes. Tight tops? There are no negative reactions. Tight bottoms? They come off and get pitched quicker than Superman can leap over a building.

You are conditioned to these responses. In "The Tyranny of Skinny, Fashion's Insider Secret" (*NYT* 3/31/02) by Kate Betts, former editor of *Harper's Bazaar* magazine, she admits participating in the obsession with thinness. She cites 1990 as a turning point with the emergence of waif-size model Kate Moss. Betts writes, "Models get skinnier and skinnier—the average model in 1985 was a size 8, while today the average model is a size 0 or 2. Yet the average American gets bigger and bigger."

This disparity in size reality is not missed by average women, and it is widely criticized. At a recent fashion show, a collaboration between *In Style* magazine and a prestigious department store, comments about the models' skeletal figures swept through the audience. We overheard a woman say, "That model is so thin, if she swallowed something you could see it go all the way down." Betts notes that while fashion can make people feel beautiful and glamorous, it can also make them feel worse if they're not as beautiful, or as thin, or as fabulous as the swans in the pictures.

Even worse, according to a series of studies directed by Dr. J. Kevin Thompson, a psychology professor at the University of South Florida, women consistently overestimate the size of their own bodies. He reports in an objective test, 95 percent of women overestimated the size of their bodies. And unlike men, women see "large" as a negative characteristic.

In a nutshell, few women see themselves as they really are.

Body image is a subjective experience. You create your body image in your mind. It is a psychological phenomenon and plays a major role in our self-concept.

Your first subjective image of yourself is created in childhood. As you grow up and age, your body changes and your mind's perception or body image adjusts. The profound and extensive biological changes associated with puberty make the body the most important aspect of the adolescent's evolving sense of self. "Who am I?" involves integrating the new physical self into a revised self-concept (see *Body Traps*, by Dr. Judith Rodin, Ph.D., 1992, William Morrow). As an adolescent you are forced to reevaluate the body image you developed as a child, and to form a new body image appropriate to the maturing self.

For example, most women recall with clarity—and often humor—buying and wearing their first bra. *"Most of my girlfriends had bras and I was so envious," said Rae. "Yet I knew when I looked in the mirror I really didn't need one. My mother saw my anxiety and marched me to a certified corsetiere, a statuesque, stern-faced woman with a measuring tape looped around her neck. After much embarrassment I emerged triumphant with a white cotton bra in size 32AA, altered smaller by two inches on each side. The next day I wore a sheer floral print blouse to show the world my achievement."*

Fawn says she made hourly alterations the day she wore her first bra. *"I stuffed it with tissue paper. After arriving at school I realized my friends were giggling about my sudden bustline, so I dashed into the girls' room and took some tissue out. It wasn't enough. I kept going back and removing more paper until it was just me and the bra."*

By your midteens, you have developed breasts, a waistline, and hips. You gaze into mirrors at your unfamiliar and changing body and check out your friends and classmates in locker rooms or at the beach. A tyranny of desired body shapes leaps at you each day from television commercials, magazines, and films. It's not surprising that teenagers are so sensitive to sociocultural norms concerning appearance.

FACT: Before puberty, girls have 10 to 15 percent more fat than boys. After puberty, girls have 20 to 30 percent more fat than boys. Boys' growth spurts involve increased muscle and lean tissue. They get tall and skinnier. Girls get curvier.

Bodies change again as girls move into their late teens and twenties because of lifestyle—either active or sedentary—and because of medications such as birth control pills. Major change is wrought by each pregnancy and childbirth. Advancing age brings menopause and bodily change as hormones ease production. Muscle mass and weight evolve, resulting in further transformation. With each physical transmutation a woman's mental self-image adjusts, often despite an intense interior dialogue of denial.

Along this journey, reality bumps up against fantasy. In the 1990s, baby boomers fiercely fought getting older. Consequently, age is not what it used to be. Older women, especially, "see themselves as generally about ten years younger than their chronological age," said David Demko, a gerontologist in Palm Beach, Florida, and the publisher of Age Venture News, a Web site for retirees. Unfortunately, this mental adjustment has not been accompanied by bodily adjustment. In truth, Americans are physically increasing in size.

"Few women see themselves as they really are."

Clothing manufacturers don't encourage clear thinking. On any given day, you can go into a department store and find pants that fit you bearing size tags ranging from size 6 to size 12. The size 6 may be from a designer firmly committed to "vanity" sizing. These companies know women love to buy clothes with single-digit size tags, even though fashion insiders are aware the brand runs one to two sizes larger. Nike, a prominent sportswear manufacturer, revised size charts in 2002 so that medium-size women of yore moved into "small" and many women formerly designated "large" suddenly fit into medium-size items. Spokespeople said the adjustment reflected their selling patterns.

Think about this next time you go shopping. You are you, not a number on a tag or category on a sign. Stop inflicting mental anguish on yourself just because a size tag reads larger than you want, or a zipper won't zip. Those size designations are no more realistic than a lot of other factors.

Two things are realistic.

1. Bottoms are the foundation of your wardrobe.

2. Because your bottom is the hardest place to fit, you need to build everything else in your wardrobe around it. Take the time to find firm base items: a well-fitting trouser, a skirt, and a short. Once you do, think in multiples. If you like the fit, the drape, the flattery of a pair of pants, for instance, buy more than one pair, and in other colors.

In chapter 6, Proportion Politics, we discussed skirts and pants for various figure types. You may wish to go back and review that information, relating it to this discussion.

LEARNING HOW TO DRESS FROM THE BOTTOMS UP

Finding pants or jeans that *really* fit is as much of a challenge as finding a new best friend when you move to a strange city. Each process is drawn out (the looking), repetitious (trying for the right fit), hopeful (looks good, maybe this one will work), and ultimately successful.

Women are conditioned to know it takes longer to find great-fitting jeans than pants. Magazines like *Jane, YM,* and *Glamour* run features once a year with banner headlines such as "We tried on 639 Jeans to Find the Right Ones for You!" or "Jeans on Trial—Each of Our Testers Tried on an Average of 43 Jeans to Find Their Favorite Fit." And theories abound, such as: (1) try on jeans lying down—which is not a useful trick in the average dressing room, (2) wash jeans in boiling hot water, or (3) put on jeans, turn the hose on them, and let them dry on you.

Pants are a different matter. Women make fateful assumptions. For example, you walk into a specialty shop and assume the size 8s with a store label will fit because you usually wear a size 8. When they don't fit, it's back to the "I've gained weight," "I ate too much last night" routine. In fact, *this store's brand of pants is not cut right for you.* They cut their pants for undernourished string beans. Go to the store next door and the store next door to that and try on their pants. Keep going until you find pants that fit so sublimely, you smile and say, "Wow." Consider buying them in every color.

BOTTOM BASICS—PANTS, JEANS, SHORTS

Pants

When selecting pants, look at construction, as certain styles will be more flattering and more comfortable for your figure type. Start with the waist. Pants come with wide waistbands, moderate one- to two-inch waistbands, bands with belt loops, and even without a waistband, cut to fit at the low point of the waistline. Generally the wider the waistband, the better they look on 75/25-body-type women with long waistlines or a 50/50 body type. A 50/50 can also wear narrow or no band pants. Women with a 25/75-body type with short waists will feel and look more balanced in pants with narrow bands or no bands.

Elastic waistbands induce trauma and controversy. Laurie, executive director of a nonprofit agency in Jackson, Mississippi, is adamant on the subject. *"I will not wear elastic anything, anywhere. It makes me feel old,"* she said. *"My mother and grandmother wore those pull-on polyester clothes. Elastic is the playground of the devil. You get larger and larger and don't even know it's happening."*

"The bottom of a woman is the hardest place to fit."

That was then, this is now. Designers today use elastic in clever, chic, and innovative ways. Eileen Fisher, Peter Nygard, St. John, Joan Vass, and David Dart design and execute wonderfully fitting clothes with elastic insets and bands. An elastic waistband on a skirt or pants, worn with a longer top over it, creates a sleek, svelte look, because the elastic allows the fabric of the bottom to move and hang evenly without pulling. The payoff is comfort you can't get in a zipped-up garment.

The next question is pleats or no pleats—and where you should wear the zipper. It depends on your figure type. In general, the best-fitting, most slimming pants are clean lined with no pockets or pleats, with a side or back zipper. If your problem is a tummy, wear any type of top that drops over your waist and stops at the hipbone.

Look carefully in the mirror and check out your image front and back if you wear lean, flat pants with a blouse or top tucked in. The whole effect will be ruined by crumples, wrinkles, or lines created by the "tucked-in culprit"—and check, too, for the dreaded VPL—visible panty line.

Banish VPL with thong panties. We know women who vow that discovering thongs "changed their life." Thongs are variously described as sexy, comfy, liberating, and visible-line free. To really be VPL-free, follow Tom Ford's advice: Gucci's *über*-designer says he goes without skivvies because it makes him feel skinnier.

You will look slimmer wearing black or other dark color bottoms, as they visually narrow your silhouette and hips. In summer, wearing a bright, pretty, solid color top with matching bottom will make you look more fetching. Slim pants in bold colored prints are eye-catching and blur the eye about exact figure proportions.

Pleats at the waistline anchor the line of pants and allow them to fall better when you put your hands into the pockets. Pants can have either a single or double pleat, and these pleats can be folded inside or out. Those folded inside give the pant a more slender appearance. Historically, the practical reason for pleats is because when one sits down, hips and buttocks have a tendency to spread and thus need space. Yes, we know: some women think pleats were put on pants to hide their tummies. They don't; quite the opposite.

It seems strange to have to say this, but pleats should *pleat* and lie flat. *Mary S., Judie's hairdresser, moaned after the holidays last year, "I've eaten so much, my pants don't pleat anymore."* Pleats actually flatter when they lie into pleats, as the folds create subtle vertical lines down the front of your body.

Pleated pants reigned supreme in the 1980s and 1990s, and then flat-front styles began reappearing. Women accustomed to the comfort and camouflage of pleated pants ignored flat-front styles as they mentally envisioned revealing their tummy pooch to the world. Cosmetics impresario Adrienne Arpel observes, "You are about thirty years old, when suddenly out pops a tummy you never had before. It's mysterious." While pleated pants seem the perfect coverage solution, try on flat-front styles as an experiment. You'll see that the less fabric there is across the stomach, the less bulk and slimmer you appear. Tunic tops, slim jackets, and over blouses lie smooth.

Pockets on pants may be decorative or intended to be functional. Classic trouser-style pockets are slanted on the seam or open on the actual seam. If you don't use pant pockets, consider stitching them shut and cutting out the pocket lining to trim your silhouette.

Most of us can use a little help to look taller, and pattern choice makes a difference. Think stripes. We're not suggesting screaming awning stripes, but rather subtle pinstripes, stripes down the side seams, and occasionally you'll find pants with solid color outer panels and inside panels of vertical stripes. Fuller-figured women should steer clear of random-size vertical stripes.

Jeans

Jeans may be the ultimate essential in your wardrobe and are the favorite of many for casual wear. Unfortunately, great-fitting jeans are often the hardest things to find. You may have to try on twenty or thirty pairs to find the perfect ones with the right detail and silhouette. Most figure types look good in a boot-cut jean with a slightly low-slung waist. Dark denims are just like black pants—you'll look thinner wearing them. To lengthen your legs, look for front vertical seaming, pinstripe patterns, or vertical panels. Wide hips are diminished visually by flare-leg styles, vertical seaming front and back, plus a low-cut waistline. Avoid jeans with a smooth back if you want to minimize the size of your butt. Instead choose jeans with well-placed pockets, yoke cuts, and vertical detail. Embellishment at the hip and waistline such as lacing, contrast yokes, or studs draw the eye and round out a boyish, straight figure.

Shorts

Shorts are a cool staple during hot weather and must-haves for golf enthusiasts, boaters, and exercisers. Yet finding the right style of short for you can be difficult. Stores and catalogs fill each spring with shorts, and unfortunately most are pleated, long, baggy, and have elastic waistlines. The prevalence of this style is *not* because it is fashionable or flattering. This style merely fits most people. It doesn't make them look good; it just fits. In the rag trade (fashion business) there is a slogan, "Get what covers the asses of the masses." Too often, women buy and wear shorts without considering alternative fit. This is one bottom style that can throw off your entire body proportion equation. Their length on your thigh, zipper placement, pocket size, and the width of the leg flare are important considerations. Pay attention and discover the short style most flattering for you!

Try a pair of those basic, baggy shorts on and look in a three-way mirror, front, back, and sideways. YUK. They add weight and bulk, making you look blocky and heavier than you are. Models wearing these styles in catalogs look great because a fashion stylist has pulled and clipped the legs in the back to make them appear slender and flattering. That is the look you want to go for.

First, try on a short that is almost knee length. Look at yourself critically and concentrate only on length. Slowly move the hem up your leg in half-inch increments until you see the best spot on your leg for your most flattering length short. Most women look best in shorts with a four-and-a-half- to five-inch inseam, as it goes over the top of the thigh and provides coverage. If you have short legs, shorter shorts make your legs look longer. Women with long legs—don't let your shorts get too long, or your legs will look short. It's goofy, but true. Avoid cuffed shorts because they wrinkle immediately and add bulk.

Now reach back and narrow the width of the short at the hemline until you see your body come into the proportion of the inverted triangle. The shoulder line should extend beyond the hip.

Next, focus on your waist. Women with a short waist will find styles with a low-slung waistband or no waistband at all are most flattering. A standard one-and-a-half- or two-inch waistband or belted styles are flattering for women with a long waist. If you want to camouflage a tummy, look for back or side zippers and a flat front.

Consider pleats in shorts the same way you treat pleats in longer pants. No pleats or stitched-down pleats are the most flattering. Pockets on the back can make your hips appear smaller, as long as the pockets are not dinky. Inset yokes in the back combined with midleg vertical seams trick the eye and make your butt appear smaller.

You'll have to look harder to find the most flattering style shorts, or you may have to pay for alterations. But you'll look and feel better, so it is worth the effort. Once you find your magic short style, buy it in multiples.

SKIRTS—THE RIGHT STYLE FOR YOU

In an era when most women favor pants of all lengths, there is definitely a place for skirts in every woman's wardrobe. Even if you love pants, we are sure you'll find a few skirts or dresses in your closet. Women who stick to skirts do it for personal reasons; they find skirts feminine, professional, or more comfortable or flattering.

Even for women who don't wear skirts very often, they are essential building blocks for your wardrobe. For casual wear, it's hard to live without a denim, navy, or khaki skirt. A basic slim black skirt is indispensable, and at least one ankle-length skirt in a solid color or pretty print is reliable for a change of pace for casual gatherings or on vacation.

Short Skirts

If you've got great legs, why not show them? Short skirts have a place in any balanced wardrobe for casual or club wear. They're great for running around town, working through errand lists, and school pickups. Many women consider short skirts necessities on vacation or for a relaxed dinner with friends at a neighborhood restaurant.

A patterned short skirt works during fall and winter with solid-colored opaque tights, while you can find an array of fun printed skirts in spring and summer. Team short skirts with sweaters or tees, and zip, you are out the door.

Skimming and Slimming Skirts

Longer skirts may be the best choices if you want to subtract a bit of your silhouette by using visual trickery. A skirt that falls in a graceful drape over your hips and is longer than it is wide makes you appear taller and slimmer. One of our favorites is a trumpet skirt, though it can be hard to find. It falls straight from the waist and flares at the hemline. Be sure it fits smoothly, without clinging, over your hips and backside. There's something about the ripple and flounce of a trumpet skirt that just makes you feel glamorous.

Circle-cut or flared skirts falling below the knee are seductive summer choices, as there is a sensuous flow and movement of sheer fabric with each sandaled step you take.

Wrap and Sarong Skirts

These are a gift from the gods to women with large bottoms. Wrap skirts create a strong, off-center vertical line, visually cutting the width of the hip. The effect is enhanced by a band print going up the "wrap" on a printed skirt. Next shopping trip, try one on and see if this works for you.

Sarong skirts work the same visual magic and pack a dose of exotic sex appeal. When men see a sarong they immediately see tropical beaches and their eyes glaze. A sarong or pareo cover-up at the beach is a gal's best friend. It hides what you want to deemphasize and looks zingy doing it. Tie an oversize scarf (about forty-five inches wide by fifty or sixty inches long) or pareo around your lower waist (just below your natural waistline) and do a loop square knot tie above the center of one leg. Push the knot lower on your body, forming a subtle angle. Now when you walk, one leg will be flashing tantalizingly and you will look sexy.

Every few years, designers such as Donna Karan come out with day-time sarong-style wrap skirts. Snap them up. You'll be glad you did.

Broomstick Skirts

We can see puzzled expressions on readers in New York City. A broomstick skirt? Women in Texas and the Southwest can't live without them. To them, they are wardrobe basics just like denim dresses. It's a cultural thing.

Broomstick skirts are ankle-length tiered skirts made of softly pleated fabric. Fans wear their broomsticks with western shirts and vests, long tunic-length sweater-knit tops, and western boots. Don't knock it until you've tried it.

Dressy Skirts

Splitting a dressy two-piece dress or suit into separate pieces could save you time, shopping, and money. Think of each piece as a separate to expand the options in your closet. For example, a lace skirt or a skirt in a fabric with a bit of shimmer looks smashing teamed with a silk charmeuse blouse or a plush sweater set. Designer Bill Blass often showed cashmere sweaters with floor-length taffeta skirts.

For dinners on the road, whether traveling or entertaining, we pack a knee-length dressy skirt in a sheer fabric with a rippling hem—either trumpet or bias cut. Wear it with your black jacket and a camisole top. Presto, you have a cocktail suit.

Skip These Skirts!

A-line skirts fairly shout dumpy, frumpy, and BORING. When you wear one everyone know that you are hiding something.

Short skirts on women with low waistlines end up looking like Band-Aids. The reason: there's more fabric up top than the minimal amount of fabric in the skirt. The skirt appears skimpy and the proportion is not flattering.

Pleated skirts are just plain tough to wear unless you are tall and slim. The best we've seen fall just below or graze the knee and have pleats stitched down over the hips. Wear it with a feminine, high-heeled shoe. At all cost, avoid resembling a lost cheerleader!

LEARN WHILE PRETENDING YOU ARE A BUYER

Throughout our book we firmly advocate dressing in separates, putting together pieces to create a variety of outfits. It's the best and most economical way to maximize everything in your closet. We automatically think mixing and matching, because as designer buyers, we had to do it for our customers. When you learn how to do it, it will give you three times as many outfits to wear with exactly the same number of items in your closet. Isn't that worth a little effort?

Here's an exercise to help.

Many women tell us they would love to be buyers for department stores or say they want to open their own women's shop. Such a career or undertaking requires a lot of hard work, education, extensive planning, and working your way up through the ranks. In this age you have to be savvier about computer applications than choosing styles, but one thing doesn't change: it takes a sense of style and a nimble mind.

Why a nimble mind? You have to learn how to mix and match parts and pieces to really be successful. As buyers we had to learn it professionally, and it's our basic philosophy for making a personal wardrobe work.

It is time to play let's pretend.

Imagine that you decide you are going to open your own shop. You want to have dresses, pants, tops and blouses, jackets, a few skirts, and maybe some suits. Dresses are easy for a store buyer. You pick out a style and color you like, figure out the sizes you want, and that's it. The nimble-mind part comes when you attack buying those pants, tops, blouses, jackets, and skirts. You can't just pick out tops *you* like, then bottoms *you* like, throw in a couple of jackets and a few skirts. Your customers would be frustrated. They want things to "go together" in their outfits. Selling a customer a pair of pants or a skirt is easy. When she says, "What do you have to go with this?" you have to have an answer. As a buyer, you anticipate your customer's taste and needs. There are questions you ask yourself before finalizing orders:

- What kinds of blouses do we need to go with the pants I selected—in what colors?
- What tees and jackets go with those skirts and shorts I selected?
- What colors, patterns, and prints do I love this season that I know my customers will want to buy from me?
- How do I figure out how many tops to buy for each bottom?
- Which styles will work for the widest array of customers?

The math is simple: there are three basic types of bottoms: skirts, pants, and shorts. There are five basic tops: jackets, blouses, shirts, tees or knit tops, and sweaters. It sounds a bit bewildering, but deciding what to order really is simple. The average sale is two to four tops for every bottom.

VISIT THE MALL—A HOMEWORK ASSIGNMENT

For experiment number two, go on an expeditionary mission to the largest mall in your area. You are not going to buy anything. This is a learning experience. Go into the misses sportswear department, regardless of what size you wear, and find sportswear groups from people such as Ralph Lauren, Jones New York, Chaus, Tommy Hilfiger, or Liz Claiborne. Notice how these groups are put together. Usually you find two styles of pants, two lengths of skirts, a knit top, a short-sleeve top and a long-sleeve option, as well as two jacket styles. Everything is executed in one color range. Most offer a solid color, two prints, a dash of stripes or graphics, or perhaps a few pieces in a textured fabric. The designers of these groups attempt to hit the taste of the widest possible range of customers. Chances are you'll find an outfit you like. Now look at the group and think of buying an outfit for your mother, a friend, or your twenty-something daughter or daughter-in-law (if you have one).

"You are you, not a number on a size tag."

Almost every season, a designer and company creates a group in black and white spiced with red or yellow. In the spring they do red, white, and blue because it always sells.

So—go back and pick out a group, and play "let's pretend" again. Select an outfit, then start expanding. Think which second top you would buy to go with your one pant. What would be your third-choice top? Now take that second top, and figure out another bottom you would like from the group.

Congratulations! You are learning how to mix and match. Now you're ready to go home and try it in your closet.

WHAT YOU LEARN IN YOUR OWN CLOSET

Oops, let's go back to the "pretend buyer" game for a moment. Every savvy clothes buyer for a department store closely examines the computer records of her merchandise sales. By tracking best-selling styles and colors, the buyer becomes smarter about what customers like and want.

You learn about your own tastes and styles by going into your closet and tracking the styles and colors of clothes you love and buy again and again. This is especially true of pants and skirts. Study your favorite bottoms and acquaint yourself with the reasons you like to wear them. Is it style? Fabric? Brand?

Bottoms are the foundation of any wardrobe. When you slip on your favorite bottoms and feel secure, comfortable, and in proportion, the rest of the pieces you wear will come together easily.

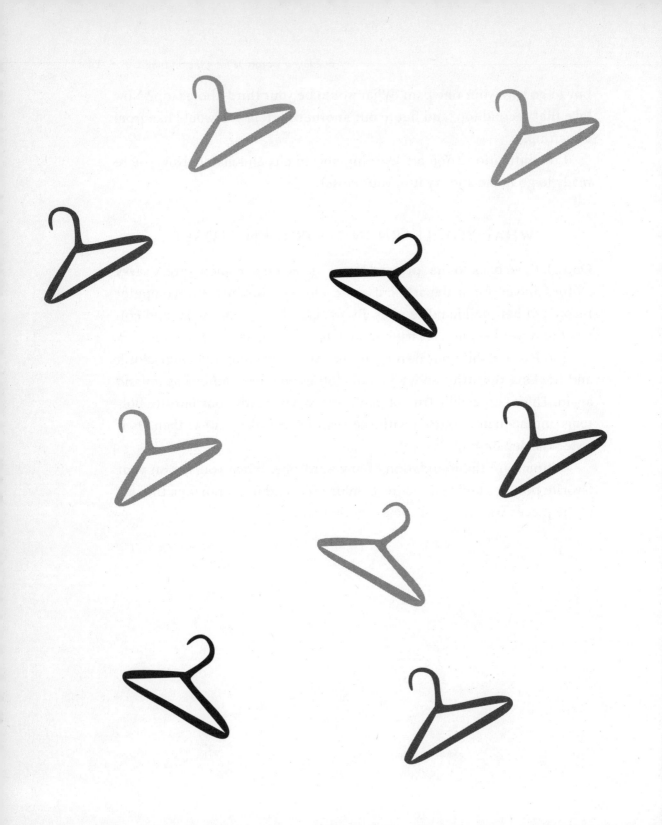

CHAPTER EIGHT

THE HIGH SIDE OF BUSINESS CASUAL

If you can't dress for success, at least dress for trying.

LYNNE ALPERT, AUTHOR
OH LORD, I SOUND JUST LIKE MAMA

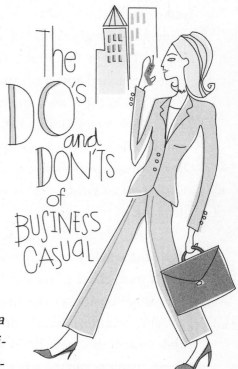

A decade ago, human resource departments had never heard of the concept of Business Casual or Corporate Casual. Out of Silicon Valley in California emerged new technologies, new ways of thinking, and a new way of dressing for business, turning over accepted traditions in modern corporate life. By 1999, the change to casual dress in America's business world had created fashion chaos.

Jennifer called Judie in desperation. "I am totally confused!" she wailed. One could understand why. Two years ago, the young woman graduated from college and joined a nationally known, extremely conservative consulting firm. Out went the jeans and tees of collegiate life, as Judie guided Jennifer's purchases toward conservative suits, shoes, and handbags.

Two years later, Jennifer got a call from an executive recruiting firm, offering her a big raise and an impressive corporate position. "Casual Fridays" were part of this allur-

ing package. Jennifer accepted and managed to limp along with her cur-rent wardrobe and a few of the weekend clothes she already had. Eight months later, the new Atlanta-based company went to casual weekdays during the summer. In the fall, the company went Business Casual every day.

Zap! Suddenly 75 percent of Jennifer's wardrobe was inappropriate. She couldn't just clear it out, though, because she still has bimonthly executive conferences at regional headquarters in Dallas and Chicago. No wonder Jennifer called Judie again with a frantic SOS. Together the two of them got down to work, as Judie helped Jennifer rethink her wardrobe for a new corporate climate.

Women have been trying to get this business-dress thing right for decades. In the 1970s, we marched into the business world in navy suits with skirts sagging at midcalf and floppy silk bow ties beneath our chins. In the 1980s an outbreak of dress-for-success consultants proclaimed power suits the ideal thing, nailing red as the ultimate power color for women. We happily eased into pantsuits and maybe bought one red jacket. Then in the 1990s, a tribe of male information types in Silicon Valley preached a new mantra: "open collars; open minds."

In truth, *these men simply didn't want to wear neckties.* For two hun-dred years, men grumbled and plotted ways to escape the tyranny of wear-ing neckties. Here it was: freedom! A giant step in men's liberation some-how—disastrously—wound up as Casual Fridays, then mutated into Business Casual, the most controversial cultural and business clothing decision of the decade.

Chairmen and CEOs, mostly male, along with human resource direc-tors (ditto, male), quickly bought into the casual idea because, hey, they didn't want to wear neckties every day either. So, swoosh, down the slip-pery slope business did slide.

The brightest minds and battalions of employees still struggle to understand this new development. We know: we marched in the front lines, giving seminars, writing articles, dispensing advice, and furnishing quotes to magazines and newspapers. Our schedules included dutifully appearing on television and attempting to define exactly what this revolution in business dress meant.

FROM THE TRENCHES OF TRAINING SEMINARS

Videotapes, rules, and new regulations spewed from thousands of seminars dedicated to defining Business Casual guidelines. Too many declared what *not* to wear. Business Casual is so ill defined, especially for women, that it results in people coming away with their own personal definition of what to wear. Thus their imaginations unleashed upon the business world amazing and dismaying concepts of what to wear in a Business Casual workplace.

A psychological tug-of-war broke out. Women wanted to participate and enjoy this new casual way of dressing, but many didn't know how to do it, and others said, "I can't afford a whole new wardrobe." Lacking the budget to buy new clothes, out came weekend wear. This confusion can result in low morale.

"I feel sloppy when I am working with my clients now," said Lydia, a graphics art consultant for a large printing company. "My self-confidence is affected and my sales have suffered. I'm dressing up again but feel out of place in the office. I'm lost. What is the answer?"

A fatal step ensued—HR (human resources) and unknown others decided that "dressing casual" in the workplace is an employee incentive. Job applicants hear enticing entreaties: "This company is a casual workplace." It is tough to make a U-turn about this type of managerial decision.

Here we are in 2003+ and still no one knows what the rules are. Simple reason: they are *indefinable*. Well, to men, that is.

Put twenty businesswomen in a room and ask them what they would wear to an *indefinable* business event, and seventeen out of the twenty would answer, "My black pantsuit."

Whereas guys would think a knit polo shirt and pleated khakis are just the ticket.

We rest our case.

Men are befuddled, in full retreat. Muffled cries echo outside executive conference rooms: "Our employees look like they are at Disney World or the airport." "We've got to do something!"

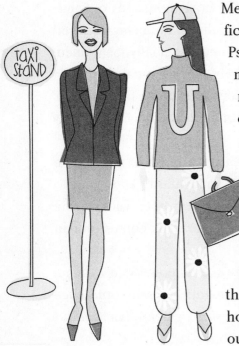

Men step up, ready to make the ultimate sacrifice, volunteering to go back to suits and *ties.* Psychological warfare is rampant. Planted media stories speculate about a return to a more formal workplace. Advertising speaks of "the return to professionalism." Male mannequins in store windows on Fifth Avenue in New York sport suits and ties. With the stock market in a continuing swoon, Wall Street CEOs heralded fall 2002 by ordering their minions back into suits—*every day.*

After work, businesswomen chuckle over their Cosmopolitans and white wine, "Ho, ho, ho! Let them go back to ties, we're staying in our black pantsuits."

IT'S A SLIGHT RELAXATION, NOT A PAJAMA PARTY

In chapter 1, The Circle of Your Life, you identified between 30 to 60 percent of your wardrobe needs as clothing for your working life. Due to the flexibility built into a wavering definition of Business Casual, you have wonderful options both to utilize your clothes for more than one category of activity, and to define your individuality and business aspirations by your appearance. Young women must be especially careful to define the differences between dressing for work and for private activities. Corporate and business environments are not appropriate venues for expressing sexuality through dress.

Despite the upheaval resulting from the arrival of Business Casual in the workplace and what has been described as the casualization of America, women rising through management ranks stick to their suits. Flip through *Fast Company, Forbes,* or the *Wall Street Journal* and pictures of notable women in government posts and CEO positions reveal a suit to be their first choice of attire. Board a plane Monday morning or on a Thursday or Friday afternoon, and professional businesswomen stand out because their appearance is polished and professional. These aircraft are usually also occupied by businessmen (an assumption, as they carry laptops) wearing pleated khaki pants and polo shirts with a company logo stitched on their chest or sleeve—just like most people wear for sponsored or PGA golf tournaments. These women know that wearing a suit conveys authority and speaks for their abilities.

Distinctions make a difference. Women sorted themselves into several categories in the "Dress for Success" era prior to Casual Fridays. Banking, consulting, and corporate businesses called for conservative dress. Marketing and service organizations took a slightly more liberal approach to formality, while creative fields such as publishing and advertising enjoyed the most freedom. Most women understand the difference between the definition of a woman with a job, and a woman with a career or career aspirations. The former requires a less "dressed-up" approach than the latter.

We believe a similar attitude and understanding of how to combine, mix, and match basic styles is key to being successful, regardless of your business situation.

The human resource director of a large Miami law firm booked Jackie for two training sessions on Business Casual dress. The director felt that the associates in direct contact with clients and the staff working behind the scenes had a divided attitude toward the subject. "Our front-of-the-house people seem to have a sense of responsibility when putting together the pieces for corporate or casual days. We feel that the other part of the staff feels that because they have no client contact, they can dress any way they want to dress. It's a real problem," she said.

Our experience as consultants with other companies in similar circumstances convinced us to mix these groups, despite differences in disposable income. It is a visible boost to the self-esteem of behind-the-scene staff members to be included as part of the plan for a company-wide push for a polished, professional image.

Under the section "A System That Works" later in this chapter, you may chart a wardrobe plan tailored for your work environment and position. Whether you are a woman who works or a woman committed to a long-term business career, the principles of dress are similar. The formula is the same.

A NEW WAY OF THINKING

The building blocks of a working woman's wardrobe must include jackets, pants, skirts, tees and tops, plus one or two dresses. If you view each suit piece separately, you'll realize the type of fabric makes a huge difference in whether it is formal, less formal, or weekend casual. Pants in wool crepe, woven wool or flannel are conservative, authoritative, and classic, while pants in a stretch twill are contemporary and less formal but still acceptable in most office environments. Khaki pants are the official fabric of Business Casual. Chambray, denim, or floral-printed fabric pants are strictly for downtime and weekends. Knit pants are rarely acceptable for any type of business wear.

Apply the same fabric guidelines to skirts and jackets.

Anne, a busy banking executive, called Jackie for a first consultation. While working out the Circle of Your Life and persona indicators, she vented about corporate dress versus Business Casual. Anne had definite ideas on how she should dress. "I am a skirt person and I always have them hemmed at the knee. For years, replacing my skirt with pants created a relaxed look in my mind. Now pants are everywhere, so how do I make it feel or look Business Casual?" Changing the fabric on just three pieces worked. She added two pairs of khaki trousers and a khaki cotton skirt. These, mixed with existing tops and casual jackets in her present wardrobe, filled the void.

"No one knows what the rules are."

Tops are trickier because they come in such a variety of styles. Knit tops in fine-quality smooth wool, fine cotton knits, or silk knits are dressy enough for use with formal components. Woven fabric shirts and blouses in silk, cotton, and blended yarn also make the grade. Sheerer knit tee tops in silk, cotton, or blends are best teamed with a jacketlike coverage piece. Smooth knit sweater sets, sweater shells, and turtlenecks are versatile and essential pieces. Sweater sets are a boon, functioning as an informal top and jacket. A tailored-style cardigan sweater may substitute in Business Casual for a jacket.

Career women maintain more of a dressed-up attitude in deciphering Casual Fridays and Business Casual, because through experience they learned a professional appearance commands respect. For women, this is a truth not confined to the workplace. Important community, legal, and personal financial meetings can be raised to a new level of professionalism and efficiency by the manner in which one presents oneself. School and community activists quickly learn to dress in suits before taking a plunge into politics.

An evolution in style now distinguishes the clothing of business-women from that of men. The decades-old, passé idea of women dressing like a man is history. In a skirted business suit, which is considered more formal and urban, the jacket now possesses softer shoulders and is subtly fitted. A silk blouse or shirt is discreet and feminine. Finishing touches could be pearls and pearl studs, a classic pump with a moderate heel, and a glossy black leather handbag, tote, or attaché. If your choice is a pantsuit, start building from the foot to set a mood. Select low-heeled faux or real reptile-textured loafers or a sleek smooth leather boot shoe. Again, you could choose a silk blouse or a silk knit tee, accessorized with a beautiful printed scarf. Coordinated trouser socks and an understated leather belt and a delicate pendant or pearl necklace all convey a businesslike demeanor without coming off as stuffy.

Your choice of business attire communicates an image of you to the world. Today more than ever, work is serious business. It is important that you project a consistent work image that is in sync with your persona, your business environment, and your aspirations.

A BUSINESS CASUAL SYSTEM THAT WORKS

The following philosophy is designed with several objectives in mind. By limiting the number of pieces, you save time selecting what you are going to wear, and you save money by getting the maximum versatility out of each piece. Mood Dressers, Trend Trackers, or Dramatic Personas may object, because these suggestions tend to be more business appropriate than overly expressive. But even in uniforms, women find ways of expressing their personalities through hairstyle, makeup, jewelry, accessories, and outerwear. Check both our Defining Details and Persona Pieces lists at the end of this chapter for tips.

First, redirect your thinking to *units* rather than *outfits.* A suit is an outfit. A skirt, a jacket, a blouse or pants are units. Each unit mixed with another unit gives you a fresh perspective—and a new outfit.

To illustrate the practicality and diversity of this system, imagine two shoppers:

I. Clare enters a sportswear department, and after hours of trying on clothes she comes to the register with four Business Casual outfits in various colors, each consisting of two pieces. She charges $400 to her credit card and goes home with eight pieces creating four looks.

    1. Navy patterned blouse + navy pants

    2. Raisin and white striped shirt + raisin skirt

    3. Brown long-sleeved shirt + brown tweed skirt

    4. Black turtleneck sweater + glen plaid pants

II. Cecily shops the same department. She finds a black jacket and pants with a tiny red pinstripe. The jacket will go with her solid black pants, a red skirt, and black jeans she already owns. Next she selects four tops: a crisp white shirt, a red silk knit tee with matching cardigan, and a black silk tee. Then she decides to add the pinstripe skirt and a print skirt with red and black in the coloration. Her eight pieces totaled $400 and she went home with more than twelve new looks—each bottom (pinstripe skirt, pinstripe pants, print skirt) can be worn with each top singly or in pairs.

    1. Pinstripe pants + pinstripe jacket

    2. Pinstripe pants + red tee

    3. Pinstripe pants + black tee + jacket

    4. Pinstripe pants + red sweater set

5. Pinstripe pants + white shirt + jacket

6. Pinstripe skirt + red sweater set

7. Pinstripe skirt + black tee layered under white shirt

8. Pinstripe skirt + white shirt + jacket

9. Pinstripe skirt + black tee + jacket

10. Print skirt + black tee

11. Print skirt + sweater set

12. Print skirt + red tee layered under white shirt

And the options continue—plus Cecily has a core wardrobe for the season. Which would you rather have: eight pieces and four outfits, or eight units and over twelve outfits?

The same formula could mix solid beige and navy units with one print skirt and shell top. You would have several sophisticated monochromatic outfits using the same color top to toe. The pieces would be: beige jacket, pants, and skirt; navy pants, navy print skirt, matching print top, beige blouse, navy sweater set.

1. Beige jacket + beige skirt + beige blouse

2. Beige jacket + beige pants + print blouse

3. Beige jacket + navy pants + beige blouse

4. Beige pants + beige blouse + navy cardigan

5. Beige pants with print tee + navy cardigan

6. Navy pants goes monochromatic + navy tee or sweater set

7. Navy pants + beige jacket worn over the navy tee

8. Navy pants + print blouse with navy cardigan

9. Beige skirt + beige blouse

10. Beige skirt + print tee

11. Beige skirt + navy tee + navy cardigan tied over shoulder
12. Print skirt + print tee
13. Print skirt + print tee + beige jacket
14. Print skirt + print tee + navy cardigan
15. Print skirt + sweater set

Additional units from our Persona Pieces list can mix with these core units, creating additional looks expressing your independent and creative point of view.

THE FINAL ANALYSIS

Cultural indicators in business remain in flux. Silicon Valley's star is dim, with bankruptcies on the rise and its influence vanquished. As the stock market languishes, prognosticators preach change, any type of change: in interest rates, technology, business dress, and values—hoping for stability.

Years have passed since the advent of Business Casual and turmoil in industry churns on. It is unlikely that management will ever be able to shift people back to neckties and pantyhose, but a shift from Business Casual up to Professional Casual

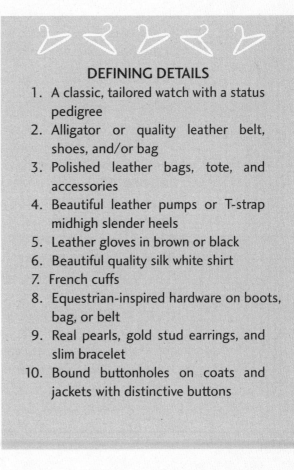

DEFINING DETAILS
1. A classic, tailored watch with a status pedigree
2. Alligator or quality leather belt, shoes, and/or bag
3. Polished leather bags, tote, and accessories
4. Beautiful leather pumps or T-strap midhigh slender heels
5. Leather gloves in brown or black
6. Beautiful quality silk white shirt
7. French cuffs
8. Equestrian-inspired hardware on boots, bag, or belt
9. Real pearls, gold stud earrings, and slim bracelet
10. Bound buttonholes on coats and jackets with distinctive buttons

PERSONA PIECES

These items are ways to express yourself while adding value and style to your working wardrobe. When teamed with upscale or weekend pieces, each piece is a "mixer" versatile enough to move from corporate to casual.

1. Menswear-inspired patterned jacket in a tweed, gun check, houndstooth, plaid, or herringbone.
2. A distinctive textured jacket such as fleece, camel hair, raw silk, or boucle
3. A fabric handbag or tote in tapestry, print, or jacquard fabric
4. Red gloves, red tee, red leather jacket, red handbag. Mix with black or gray pieces.
5. A colorful silk scarf with your suit or a long, oblong knit scarf and cap with your winter coat
6. Richly colored yet conservative print or patterned trouser socks
7. Flattering and distinctive eyeglass frames and sunglasses
8. An oversize wool wrap to fling over your coat in a rich print or a striking black-and-white tweed or houndstooth print
9. Elegant leather gloves, wallet, cosmetic case, cell phone case
10. Signature cuff bracelets in real gold or silver. Chunky and bold or small and subtle necklaces and earrings in expressive semiprecious stones or cultured pearls
11. Distinctive print, plaid, or other conservatively patterned umbrella
12. Unusual or offbeat color combinations such as pale blue and coffee brown, coral and gray, aqua and forest green, lavender and navy, purple and red
13. A mixable print or patterned skirt in a black and white tiny dot, large plaid, or three to four color geometric print
14. Suede, leather, or leather-trimmed topper jacket
15. Beautiful lace lingerie in flattering colors

is likely. *The decision you must make is a personal one expressing your own ambitions and course for the future.* People form impressions about you within seconds of meeting and seeing you. The message you send is your decision. But to look smart and professional, you need not return to the old concept of power suits. By working within a loose framework of traditional forms you can relax the formality without losing the psychological impression of competence, adeptness, and authority. You are likely to be noticed, command respect, and—more important—feel confident.

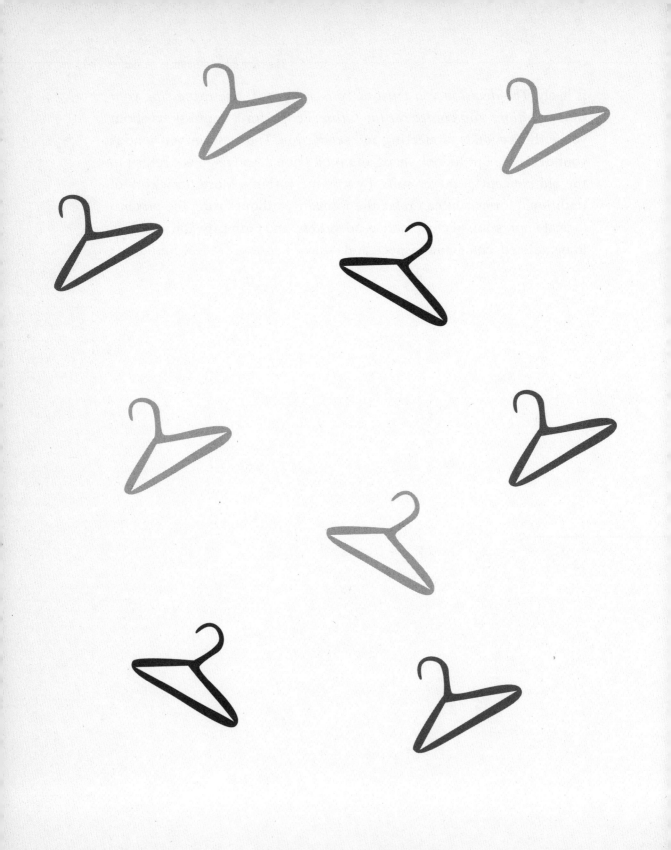

CHAPTER NINE

LET'S GO SHOPPING!

I'm not obsessed with clothes but I do understand
"retail therapy."

RANIA, QUEEN OF JORDAN

As women, we all understand and relate to the concept of retail therapy. Men just do not get it. One fellow we know thought when his wife mentioned retail therapy that she was going to install a couch in the closet. Males have a phobia about shopping; mention a trip to the mall together and watch his anxiety rocket.

Retail therapy for women is self-medication for the soul, a key ingredient of our emotional history, a stress buster, a soothing means of meditation. Women go shopping because it makes them feel better. It transforms them internally. *"I am so depressed I am going shopping,"* said Marjorie. *"I just got a raise, I'm going shopping to celebrate,"* says Dana. *"I've got to get out of this house. I'm going shopping,"* said Tina.

Why do *you* go clothes shopping? Seriously, what motivates you? Of course you shop out of need, for a new season, replacements, or a special event. Do you also occasionally shop out of boredom or for disengagement? Do you head to the mall looking for something that's missing in your life? Is spending money a manifestation of a problem in your emotional psyche?

Beverly and Alix, high-powered businesswomen we met in Boston, say they shop after work as a diversion. *"I love to wander down a mall and look at window displays or go into stores and study mannequins and experiment with new products. My job keeps me in a pressure cooker all day. Shopping helps break the stress,"* said Beverly.

These women are not alone. Each fall, stores brace for an onslaught of mothers shopping alone the week after primary school begins. It's a freedom rite, after long summer days spent tending their children.

Dorothy, a business consultant with clients on three continents, depends upon Jackie during four major preseason shopping excursions annually. For years, the team goal is to buy everything Dorothy will need for the coming three months. Yet each time they take inventory before departing, new items have magically appeared in Dorothy's closet. *"Jackie, you remember these. We bought them together," said her client. Jackie knew she had never seen the clothes before. Once, Dorothy's daughter witnessed the routine and started laughing. "Mom, you are a flagrant fib teller. Jackie, don't you know that Mom goes shopping without you? It's not about the clothes. It's about the hunt. She doesn't want to give up the rush she gets from finding a super bargain or a fabulous dress by accident." Dorothy is an arousal type, a thrill seeker. She is addicted to that euphoric rush.*

Perhaps you, too, shop for the hunt and the rush. Or are you an emulator?

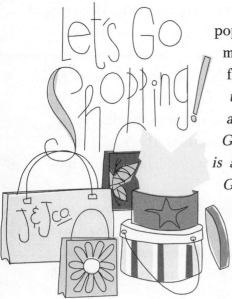

Young women sometimes fixate on current pop stars and adopt a singer's style of dress, makeup, or hairstyle. Other women admire a film star's or celebrity's style. *Gerri, a statuesque model type, adores Nicole Kidman and her adventurous flair. "Oh, my gosh,"* Gerri shrieked in a store recently. *"This dress is an exact copy of what Nicole wore to the Golden Globes. I've got to try it on."* And into the dressing room she went.

Chris, a film addict, summoned Jackie because "I made a very expensive mistake. You've got to help me." The previous evening she had watched The Prince of

Tides, *starring Barbra Streisand. "I thought I was Barbra. I thought I was her character in those sleek, elegant suits." That morning on a quick business trip, Chris passed a factory outlet mall, stopped, and bought three look-alike suits, "all marked down 65 percent in a designer outlet. That made it even better," she said. Late that night, Chris tried them on at home and realized, "I am not Barbra. I am not even close." While beautiful, the suits did not fit and were not for her body proportions or fash-ion persona. Worse, they were stamped FINAL SALE—NOT RETURN-ABLE. They arrived in a consignment store bearing the original price tickets.*

> **"Part of knowing yourself is understanding your 'price points.'"**

Markdowns and sales can turn women's brains off. At full price two months ago, Ruth thought a dress was ugly. At 66 percent off regular price, she scoops it up. Did it magically get prettier? What is it about get-ting a bargain that kicks our emotions into high gear?

Maggie and Betty know every store within 150 miles of their home in Akron, Ohio, and when each one is having a sale. "Shopping for bargains is a time-honored excuse to go shopping," says Betty. Snaring a bargain is exhilarating—and habit forming. Once you land one, chances are you go back again and again, trying to find more.

Several discount stores grew into national chains by sprinkling hid-den superbuys throughout their stores. One buyer for such a store calls her special bargains "fish food."

THE "I HATE TO SHOP" EPIDEMIC

Alas, in recent years, shopping as therapy is failing because of conflict issues.

"Shopping for clothes today is just too bewildering," said Susanna. "I

wear a size 10 and wanted to buy a pantsuit to wear to the office. Last night after work I went to my favorite department store, and I had to look in seven different departments on two floors. I couldn't find a salesperson to help me find a right department or answer my questions. At one point I found something I wanted to try on, and then couldn't find a fitting room. It was exhausting. I gave up and went home."

Stores seem to be designed as mazes. Through the years, retail executives drifted from displaying merchandise by categories, such as dresses, sportswear, and athletic gear, to a lifestyle concept, such as contemporary, weekend dressing, and business. Then it was size categories such as petite, missy, women's, and plus-sizes.

Additional hassles result as merchants cling to budget categories, splitting merchandise arrangements finer. Thus you find store directories listing budget sportswear, moderate sportswear, better sportswear, bridge sportswear, and designer sportswear.

To complicate matters further, vendors such as Jones New York, Liz Claiborne, Ralph Lauren, and Tommy Hilfiger jump in, insisting on departments carrying *only* their merchandise. Each of these "brand name" areas offers casual sportswear, upscale casual sportswear, tailored separates, and dresses. All this makes sense to retail executives and vendors. But this conglomeration of choices is mass confusion and frustration for customers.

A final blow is a habit that stores just can't seem to break. If business slumps for a few days, they have two explanations: the advertising's bad or the department (or entire floor) isn't arranged correctly. *Move the merch* is retail talk for moving everything around. Yesterday you tried on a dress you were not convinced you should buy. Today you came back to get it and the place looks like a different store. Nothing—departments, racks, displays, even personnel—is where it was yesterday.

In the 1980s and 1990s, psychologists linked major life events to stress and illness and developed a chart designed to give events, such as a partner's death or moving to a new city, points. If you racked up *x* number of points in one year or six months, it was an indicator you would probably become ill. In 1991 a research team, Kohn, Lafreniere, and Gutevich, reported that hassles—defined as small, irritating, frustrating events in our daily lives—were better predictors of psychological problems such as anxiety, tensions, and worries. Waiting in line, finding a parking place, locating a desired product, being stuck in traffic—all are considered to be frustrations which can create a proclivity for illness.

Buying a pair of black pants could well be used as a typical hassle in such a study. Today, to find those pants, a woman has to shop four to seven different areas, and several floors of an average department store. Then finding a sales associate to ring up your

"You don't have to look at everything to find what you need."

purchase is a major challenge. Often when you can find an associate she is ill informed, untrained, or both. Customer service is so bad, an August 1999 Yankelovich Monitor survey reported that 53 percent of shoppers said they were willing to pay more for better service.

Are you ready to push a shopping cart around your favorite department store? Trade rumors indicate a major nationwide chain is considering this. Visualize getting a shopping cart into the average dressing room area. Ghastly.

ATTACKING DYSFUNCTIONAL SHOPPING EMPORIUMS

Curl up with a cup of coffee and listen to our revelations garnered from hundreds of dressing rooms, interviews with salespeople, and shoppers across the country! As veterans of the retail business, catalog creation, marketing, consulting (we got paid to shop malls all over the country), and fashion reportage, as well as personal shopping, we know the ins and outs of how to navigate catalogs, store racks, and shopping sites on the

Internet. We're here with insider information to help you crack the code of store layouts, the size maze, and how to become laser shoppers.

Your budget, lifestyle, fashion persona, and brand preferences are vital pieces of information you need before navigating the maze of modern shopping and taking control of the experience. You may want to go back and review chapter 1, The Circle of Your Life; the analysis of your fashion persona in chapter 4; and guidelines for your proportions in Proportion Politics, chapter 6. Doing this self-exploration is a significant timesaver and will enable you to become an efficient laser shopper.

Part of knowing yourself is understanding your "price points." Each person has a set of "price points" firmly planted in the subconscious. Your points are a series of prices you are willing to pay for specific items or objects. These vary widely from one individual to the next because of one's perceived value of these items. Your perceived value may be based on quality, comfort, status, or economical reality.

Occasionally a person has widely varying price points and concepts about perceived values.

Alex, an investment executive, has a closet full of pricey designer suits. "The fit, fabric, and workmanship are amazing in these suits. I feel powerful and confident wearing them," she said. "I wear them with tee shirts from the Gap. I buy ten at a time, five white shirts and five black shirts. Spending hundreds of dollars on tees, just because they are from designers, is crazy. The Gap makes great tee shirts."

Retail store owners and manufacturers are acutely aware of and sensitive to consumers' price points. In large department stores, buyers define their buying responsibilities by price points. For example, a dress buyer may be limited to buying dresses selling in a range from $69 to $130. Each category is arranged by price points such as budget dresses, moderate dresses, better dresses, and perhaps designer dresses. If you don't feel comfortable spending more than $100 to purchase a dress, you would be considered a "moderate" customer. Your personal price points define you as a particular type of customer in the mind-set of retailers and assist you in predetermining what areas of a store you will visit.

Inflation propels price points upward, and you may find yourself paying $5 or $10 more this year for a blouse, or you may refuse to budge your price plateau and shift to another brand, department, or store.

Before leaving home, decide what you want/need. Step one is to analyze the existing clothes in your closet. See what ingredients are missing and make a list on a three-by-five card that you can carry in your handbag. Shopping with a list is a form of self-regulation, a means of internalizing your intentions. Now imagine what you want to find. For example: is it a romantic floral dress or a club-smart *Sex and the City* look? Set a limit on how much you can/will spend and think carefully about what stores might have what you need. Plan your itinerary around their locations. Add this to your list.

> This is how I shop for bras. I go to Bloomingdale's to the fourth floor. I go there for two hours and I buy two thousand of the black, two thousand of the beige, two thousand of the white. And I ship them around between the homes and the boat and that's the end of it for maybe half a year, when I have to do it all over again.
>
> IVANA TRUMP, AUTHOR AND DESIGNER

Here is a priceless secret: you don't have to look at everything to find what you need. Because of what you've learned about yourself, you know that only a small percent of what is in a store or in a mall is "you."

In chapter 1, The Circle of Your Life, Becky realized that shifting from full-time to part-time work completely changed her wardrobe needs. Though she had suits for visiting clients, Becky also needed more casual outfits to wear while working at home or participating in suburban community activities. In chapter 4, Becky discovered her persona split between Natural and Modernist. Her tendency toward tracking trends dissipated after the birth of Justin, her second child. Proportion Politics revealed she has a low waist. *"I never knew that before. At last I understand why nothing is ever long enough to fit my upper body length. Now I buy 'tall' tops whenever I can find them or just have to look at a tee to know whether it will fit me,"* she said. And she now looks for swimwear labeled *"long torso."*

In cleaning out her closet, Becky learned she gravitates toward three favorite brands of sportswear because they fit her body well. And she knows what style or silhouette of dress designs works for her taste level, lifestyle, and proportions, without having to try on half the suits and dresses on a rack. Our young mother also noticed she reaches for two outfits repeatedly, so she decided to buy several more with the same cut and fit. Armed with this knowledge, Becky is well on her way to becoming a black belt shopper.

Take what you have learned about yourself and put it in the top of your consciousness. When you go out shopping in the future, do it with purpose and direction. Use a kind of tunnel vision, tuning out departments or stores you know will not have anything of interest to you because of their attitude/target customer, cost, size specialty, and brand selection.

> Don't go making purchases instead of fixing your life.
>
> RENÉE ZELLWEGER, ACTOR

In new stores or a store you haven't visited in a while, try our circle scan. We use it in New York City, as stores there constantly morph and change in department layout and designer name boutiques. First we study a store plan, narrowing down which floors we think we want to shop. Then we go to those floors and make a circle loop around each floor, noting areas of interest by assessing displays and clothing racks at the front of the departments. If we relate to what we see, we mentally tag it as interesting and keep going around. On a second loop we slowly visit each department noted, and start shopping.

Specialty stores resemble garden plots overgrown with crisscross X racks. Each rack is festooned with mix-and-match looks. Wander down and around several rows of racks and see if the items featured appeal to you. If you are interested, keep looking and shopping. If not, beat a fast exit.

SIZE WISE SAVVY

During a visit to Yesterdaze, a vintage store for fashion and collectibles, Judie overheard the owner instructing a customer: "In 1950s and 1960s clothing you will have to go up several sizes from what you wear today, because sizes back then were smaller than they are today. For instance, if you wore a size 20 then, you will wear a 14 today." Yikes, that means a size 6 then would be a size 0 today!

It reminded us of an anecdote we heard about a woman's first visit abroad. When seeing European sizes, Barbara said, "I have always wanted to have a larger bust and was delighted to learn I was a size 44 in France."

How did we ever get to be so controlled by that tiny number sewn into every garment we buy? We see women who are fanatical about never wearing anything larger than a size 6 or 8 or 10. It is crazy. As you learned in chapter 6, Proportion Politics, it is not about size anyway, it is about proportion. Need evidence? The reason the selection in dress departments keeps getting smaller is because most women wear different sizes on the top and bottom of their bodies, forcing them to buy separates, not dresses.

Broad ranges of sizes are used, such as petite, misses, women's, and tall. Petite sizes are proportioned for women four feet eleven inches tall to five feet three inches tall, sizes 0 to 14. Misses or missy sizes are for

women five feet four inches to five feet seven inches
tall for sizes 2 to 16. Women's sizes range from sizes
14W to 28W, for women who are five feet four
inches tall to five feet seven inches tall. Women-
size clothing averages one to two inches larger
than a missy size. For example: a missy size 14 or 16
skirt is approximately two inches narrower
in width than a women's size 14W or
16W skirt. Tall sizes are proportioned to
women five feet eight inches to six feet,
with sleeves, body length, and inseams
cut longer. Young women from junior
high school until their early twenties wear
junior sizes ranging from 1 to 13, running in odd numbers (3, 5, 7, 9, 11).

So there you have it, except for the exceptions. Among those are
women with short waists fitting into petite tops, or women with long legs
fitting into tall pants regardless of their height.

Do not let size dictate to you. Take size mania out of your shopping
experience and replace it with a dedication to finding clothes that fit
your wonderful, unique body.

TRUE TALES OF SALE-RACK PHILOSOPHY AND SUCCESS

Sale racks make women emotional. You get revved about finding style
first, instead of substance or basics. We have a new mantra for you: It's just
as easy to buy something you love, need, and want on sale, as it is to go
home with an iffy impulsive purchase. Use sales to stock up on basics: a
black suit, white shirt, twin sweater set, slim brown skirt, cotton tee tops.
They are all there at 50 percent off or more. These are not the most exciting pieces, but you'll love them each time you reach for one to finish an
outfit.

Before leaving home, look through newspaper inserts, mailers, and advertisements for discount coupons. Cut them out and tuck them in your wallet. A coupon reading "$5 off any purchase of $15 or more" is like cash. If a coupon reads "20% off a single purchase" save it for a big-ticket item. Highlight expiration dates and plan accordingly. Stores may offer an early bird saving, say 25 percent off purchases between 7 A.M. to 9 A.M. If you are a morning person, go for it. You'll beat the crowds and save money.

Here is your strategy: when you enter a shop or department during a sale, always look around carefully. Way in the back is where the BIG bargains lurk. Start at the rack with 75 percent off. Look for basics first and snatch them up. If part of your mission is finding a match-up piece, such as a blouse for your gray suit, take the suit with you and see what you can find that fills the bill. Move to the rack that is 66 percent off, repeat the process, then hit the 50 percent off selection and do it again.

You may spot items that make you think, "I really love that." Go ahead, put it on hold, or hang it last on the rack by the next highest size doughnut, those plastic rings with sizes printed on them. It's like your own personal hold rack. In highly competitive situations, grab and hold on to what you think are "maybes." After you have worked all the racks for basics and match-up pieces, cruise back and check out whether you still really like what caught your fancy on your first pass.

Pay special attention to signs on walls and over racks. Especially note when they indicate a markdown to be taken at checkout. Not marking price tags is a lazy way for the store to cut down on work for personnel. To confirm the cut in price, look for a courtesy bar code reader in the area or ask an associate to confirm the discounted price. When checking out, say, "A sign indicated a markdown. What is my actual purchase price?" before they ring it up. Several times, we have been amazed to discover that *additional* computer markdowns took our purchase price down even further.

Do a visual check to see if you think something marked in your size range *really* looks like it is that size. Many things languish unsold during their regular season because they are labeled incorrectly. If you suspect this is the case, try on one size up or another size down to be double sure.

Okay, maybe you're getting grumpy, thinking, "I'm just going to buy something I want and I don't care if these two don't like it." Go ahead, reward yourself! Just be sure you love it, you have something to wear it with, and you feel great in it.

Be wary of buying heart thumpers: hip, hot fashion items with big markdowns and limited wear life. Trendy clothes are like fresh produce— great when fresh, icky and useless after too long.

"Sale racks make women emotional. Ask yourself, 'Would I buy this at regular price if I could have afforded it?'"

A shopping-dependent crew in San Antonio, Texas, believes four heads are better than one when shopping. With the cunning of General Schwarzkopf, their leader Angie organizes bimonthly shopping trips. They set dates based on inside knowledge gleaned from store associates, meet for a car pool at 7:30 A.M., double-check coupons, and head out, visiting *every* branch of a store chain staging a sale. Twice a year, their destination is Dallas. Of course they have a blast, and you could too.

SALE TIPS: MAKING EVERY DOLLAR COUNT

Prior to sale shopping, look around at the new arrivals, trendy items for the coming season. Note styles, colors, and designs. We bet you will find similar items on the sale rack. Buyers test new-trend looks and often are ahead of customer awareness. Since most stores follow set markdown calendars, these test items go on sale before a trend is established.

Before paying for any sale item, ask yourself, "Would I have bought this at regular price if I could have afforded it?" If the answer is yes, it's a good buy. If the answer is no, put it back on the rack.

Find more tips on sale strategies in our book end bonus, "Fifty Hot Tips."

SEASONAL FASHION CALENDAR

Fashion cycles make no sense whatsoever, but you can't fight it. Winter coats are in stores in summer; swimsuits pop up in December along with flowered capri pants. Coats go on sale in October, and swimsuits are marked down in early May, just about the time you want to buy one. Don't these store people know they could make more money by waiting? Well, yes, they do. But stores are competitive, and each one wants to be first to lure you in. Once upon a time, all swimwear got marked down July Fourth and women waited for the event. Store A decided, "Aha, let's mark down swimsuits in late June and beat everyone else." Naturally store B followed, moving their markdown date a week before Store A. The final analysis: if you wait until you need something, chances are it will be gone.

Shop outlet stores at season's end to find wear-now clothing needs. For example, in late July and early August you can still find summer clothes at outlets, because stores move their end-of-season leftovers to these locations.

In the beginning of fashion time, a guru decreed that women wanted to shop ahead. Take note of these seasonal guidelines to help you get the choice of each season's crop. If you are hard to fit or need a different size jacket from the size of your skirt or pant, go early in the season for the best selection.

Unless you live in the Sunbelt, never ever plan a shopping spree in January, and for heaven's sake don't let your club or organization even THINK about staging a fashion show in January. Stores let their stocks dwindle after the holidays in preparation for inventory mid-month. The less merchandise stores have to count, the faster the inventory goes.

Shopping for spring? Stores in sunny climes are often used for testing merchandise, so if you live in the Sunbelt, you need to shop in early February. Up north, spring shoppers had best start nibbling in late

February and get the best of the season in March. Stores that are down south, especially in Florida, get a Preview Season of swimwear early in the year. Big swimsuit manufacturers use Preview to predict selling patterns during the normal swimsuit season.

Late March and early April heralds the arrival of summer clothes. Get out there and buy that swimsuit!

By June, the summer fashion season is over. You will find bits and pieces; you'll have trouble finding your size and choice in color.

July is preseason sale time. Stores tempt you with limited-time-only sale prices on fall merchandise. It's a good opportunity to stock up on basics and snap up transitional clothes for early fall.

Even with the mercury soaring to the nineties in August, go shopping NOW for fall. Mid-to-late August and early September is peak selection period.

Heavy woolens, plush plaids, and cashmere sweaters hit stores in October. With holiday season around the corner, watch for festive clothing late in the month.

In early November, nail special-occasion clothes for Thanksgiving and beyond. By December you'll find only sequins on the floor.

I'm also just a girl and I like to shop.

GWYNETH PALTROW, ACTOR

RETURN POLICIES

You get a purchase home, and it hits you—I can't afford this, the color is wrong, it looked different in the store's fluorescent lights, my guy hates it on me, or what was I thinking? We've all suffered it. Buyer's remorse prompts store returns. The key is to act promptly. *Return merchandise as soon as you possibly can do it.*

Be certain you know a company's or store's return policy before you purchase anything. If you don't know it, ask what it is. Be aware of time limits and refund specifications, such as store credit only or credit card credit only or no cash refunds. Waiting thirty, sixty, or ninety days for a store to send you a check reimbursement may be a financial hardship. Women tell us this is a part of shopping they find most intimidating. It's withering to attempt to return something only to be told "we have a thirty-day return limit policy" and you missed it by two days.

When making a return, be direct and quietly assertive. *Have your sales receipt ready.* State clearly, "I need to return this and get a refund or credit because _____ (state reason)." This is a business transaction, not a personal assault on your self-esteem. Most stores are happy to accommodate, provided you have a receipt and meet the return-time limits. Occasionally you might be challenged. Answer questions without getting upset and patiently wait if "a manager has to okay this." The wait is worth getting your money back. If you insist on attempting a refund or credit without a receipt or past the time limit, be ready to accept the consequences, which usually is less than full credit or no return at all. If you've been away for six weeks be contrite, apologize, and go for sympathy.

Some women are habitual returners, though they're rare. Every seasoned salesperson knows a customer who returns almost everything she buys. Such behavior is hard to understand, as it wastes vast amounts of time. When these women darken the door of a store or department, salespeople dive for cover. If you return many of your purchases it is worthwhile to consider your motivations:

first in buying, then in returning. Is it indecision? Is it a bid for attention? Is it a simple mistake you repeat too often?

SIX KEYS TO BECOMING A LASER SHOPPER

1. Know yourself. Keep in mind your budget, lifestyle, fashion persona, sizes, most flattering silhouettes, and favorite brands.

2. Shop with a list. Establish a list near your closet and keep tabs on what you need to buy and what needs repair.

3. Plan your shopping trip ahead. Check for sales, coupons, and special value buys. Plan your itinerary so you get where you need to go before you become exhausted looking in the wrong places.

4. Shop with a purpose, focusing on merchandise for you. Narrow your shopping to appropriate stores and departments within your budget and taste level.

5. Browse shops at the beginning of each season, just before a sale, or for pleasurable distraction. Notice if a style or fabric pattern appears in two, three, or more stores. Even if you love it, you will want to pass—unless you want to see lots of other women wearing the same thing that you are.

6. Know return policies.

TRAVEL STOPS AND TREND RERUNS

Everyone likes to shop when they travel. Be especially aware of seasonal bonanzas. For example, San Francisco is a gold mine of marked-down spring and summer clothing for visitors from Sunbelt states. In northern California, it never gets really warm enough for women to buy large spring/summer wardrobes. The reverse is true in Florida. People from northern states find good selections on fall and winter markdowns, as weather in Florida rarely drops below fifty degrees.

Don't get in a rut by buying more of what you already have, unless it's a wardrobe building block such as a black pantsuit. Even then, consider a different collar style, an updated detail, or more interesting fabric.

Lost loves rediscovered can disappoint us. Karin told us of the thrill she felt when designer Diane Von Furstenberg brought back her fabled wrap dresses in the late 1990s. *"I loved those dresses back when she became famous for their style. After seeing a business story about Diane's comeback, I tracked down a store carrying her new line. I took three dresses into a fitting room, slipped into one, and turned to the mirror. I looked dreadful. The body I live in now is NOT the body I had in 1973."*

Young fashion magazine assistants came up with an axiom about recycled trends. "If you wore this trend the first time around, DON'T even think about trying to wear it this time." But according to Judith Krantz— a best-selling author, fashion fanatic, and woman of a certain age—just like love, the second time around for a trend is lovelier. *"If I didn't wear trends on the second or third time around, I'd be walking around naked."*

CRUISING CATALOGS AND SHOPPING ON THE INTERNET: HAZARDS AND BENEFITS

Each day, millions of catalogs fill mailboxes across the United States. Buy from one, and three new ones soon arrive. For many time-starved women, flipping through catalogs is their retail therapy. In a sense, the experience is more rewarding than visiting a real store. There's color, attitude, atmosphere, beautiful models, entertaining descriptions, and sharp photography. All entice the reader/shopper into ordering. Active sportswear for running, exercising, or jogging ordered out of a catalog filled with pictures of cliff-clutching rock climbers and skiers cutting down untouched mountain peaks assures authenticity in the seriousness of the sport gear offered. Another catalog sells serenity and ease, with models dreamily strolling beaches, pensively staring out to sea from deserted dunes, and meditating in windswept meadows. They imply a dollop of peacefulness in every UPS delivery from this source.

The most successful catalogs are expressions of carefully constructed concepts. Marketers focus on a customer type or niche, lifestyle, taste trend, or activity, and present the merchandise enhanced with settings, presentation, models, and props appropriate to the key concept.

As you sort through your catalogs, you make decisions based on how much you identify with the persona illustrated in each one. Some catalogs go directly into trash cans while others are carefully perused. Collect a week's worth of catalogs from your mailbox, sort them, and see if each one you retain matches your fashion persona and/or the Circle of Your Life activities.

Catalogs and Internet sites add additional challenges to your shopping skills. You make decisions without knowing exact colors, fit, or the tactile feel of fabrics. Study the pictures of desired products. While most catalog producers strive for accuracy in color reproduction, it can be distorted. Read copy carefully for additional descriptive help and specifics such as type of cotton, distressed finishes, Lycra content, length of garment, and especially fit. Fit varies dramatically from one catalog to another. It is important to study size charts and match your "just-measured dimensions" to those on the chart. Recently we've noted catalogs adding an additional size chart, a "Modern" chart in addition to the standard misses and women's size charts. Modern sizes are on the small side, $\frac{1}{4}$ to $1\frac{1}{2}$ inches in variance from the others. A few catalogs illustrate figure drawings with exact fitting instructions, plus an explanation of terms such as "loose fit," "drop waist," "slim fit," and waistband height. The array of waistband fitting schemes is vast. If you still are unsure about a description, call and ask a customer representative.

It is imperative that you study shipping charges in catalogs carefully. It is a profit-making aspect of the business; most shipping charges defy logic and many are outlandishly expensive, considering the item shipped. Take into account the convenience and time saved, but also the second shipping charge of possible returns.

Returns of mail order and Internet orders can be quite complex. Before ordering, study each company's rules and regulations. Again, the variation of accommodation and lack of it is mind-boggling. Returned items do get lost in transit, and you, not the company, are most likely to suffer the consequences.

That said, we admit we love shopping from catalogs and on the Internet, especially at busy times of the year. In a country with only 225 cities with population over 100,000 (*American Demographics* 8/02), Internet and catalog shopping opens up worlds of choices not usually available at home to many people.

Ah, and quick catalog ordering on the Internet is a psychological boon. Shopping this way gives you instant gratification. You see it, you want it, and in a few strokes, it is yours—at least in a few shipping days!

LET'S GO SHOPPING—A QUIZ FOR YOU

In this chapter, we discussed price points and perceived value. To help you understand your personal attitudes and limits regarding shopping, take a few minutes and review the following questions. See if you come up with a pattern in your shopping habits.

- Do you have a certain top price limit you will spend for shoes? What is it? _____ What would be an exception to your rule?_____

- Do you stay in a specific price range when shopping for a handbag? What is it?_____ What qualities would make you go over this limit?_____

- Do you have price point limits when purchasing:
    - A sportswear jacket? What is it?_____
    - Pants? _____
    - Suit? _____
    - Blouse? _____
    - Skirt? _____
    - Coat? _____
- Is there a category you feel you indulge in, out of proportion to your price plateau for other items?
    - What? _____
    - Why? _____
- What are three of your favorite stores? _____
  _____
- What are three of your favorite brands? _____
  _____
- What brand do you buy that you consider a splurge?
  _____
- Do you shop out of need, for distraction or for entertainment, or for social or emotional reasons? _____
  _____
- Do you collect and save shopping bags from chic stores?
  _____
- Do you buy for style or price? What do you put first as a consideration when shopping? _____
- What two reasons would make you pay full price for an item?
  _____
- Do you consider fabric quality when purchasing clothes?
  _____

- Are you willing to purchase any size if it looks great on you?

  _____

- What is your favorite mall or shopping area?_____

  _____

  - Is it upscale? _____

  - Discount?_____

  - Outlet?_____

Overall, can you reach any conclusions about what your motivations are when shopping?

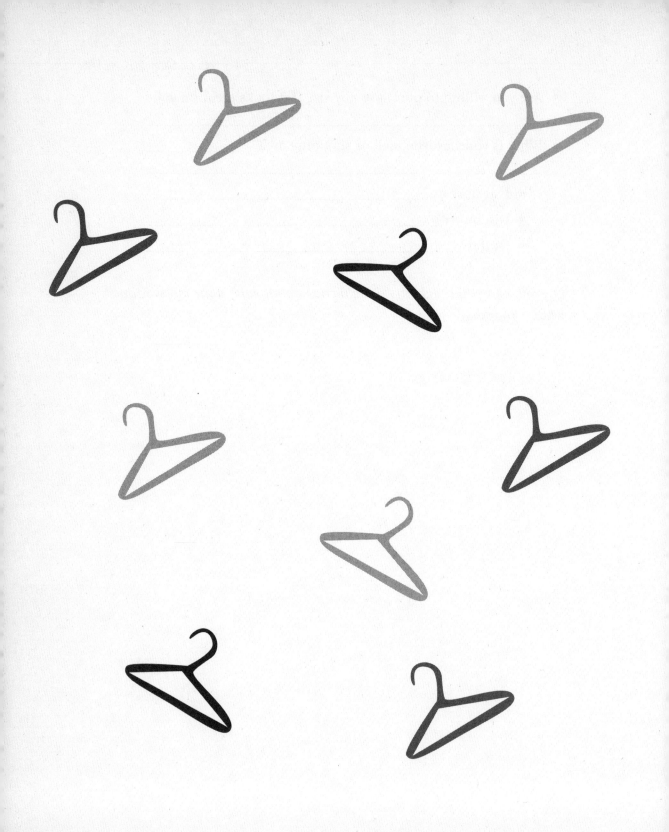

CHAPTER TEN

PUNCH PIECES AND FINISHING TOUCHES

Clothes without accessories are like sex without an orgasm.

ROBERT LEE MORRIS, JEWELRY DESIGNER

Gilding your fashion persona with shoes, handbags, jewelry, and such are surefire clues to the real you. Accessories define or communicate your fashion persona, they add character and enhance your image. Accessories can set a mood, send a signal, entice. They tip others to who you are—your daring, conservatism, status, and sexuality, even your sense of humor. Accessories are the magicians in your closet. A change of shoes, handbag, and jewelry transforms a suit for the office into a suit for a night on the town.

Accessories add interest; they embellish and articulate your persona while enhancing positive aspects of your appearance. With these details you subtly add quality and finish, as well as a focal point. A focal point accessory might be a beautiful shoe, an unusual handbag, or perhaps a striking necklace, earrings, or a pin.

When accessorizing, it is important to consider scale and balance. Too little or the same thing each day is boring, while too much is distracting. For many women, accessories are the hardest things to do. They are difficult because their eye doesn't allow them to see each piece as an integral part of the whole. If you suffer this malady, think of accessories as details you add to your overall impression. Too much zing, zing and the eye goes bump, bump, bump when it sees you. Add too

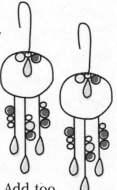

little and it is like an empty white room with no windows and no interesting point of focus. Add detail/accessories with restraint, like cooking with spice. You want to enhance, not overwhelm.

Only seasoned fashion designers such as Oscar de la Renta or highly skilled interior designers such as Mario Buatta are capable of pulling off a look blending flamboyant colors, multicolored prints, swirls, swags, flowing fabrics, and multiple clusters of accessories in one outfit or one room. Ask your mirror reflection, "Can I see myself or do I see my stuff?"

WHY YOU CHOOSE AND WEAR THEM

Your interest in accessories rises and falls during yearly fashion cycles. *"Women buy accessories when not much creatively is happening in fashion,"* says our friend Sydney, who does trend tracking for a marketing firm. *"And for many years, full-figured women in upper economic brackets bought fabulous bags, shoes, and gold jewelry because they couldn't spend money on clothes. Manufacturers ignored these women as a segment of the fashion market."*

The real beauty of accessories is that you can take some risks on new ideas and experiment without going broke. Women indulge in what they can afford or what fits. *Georgia, a style-struck supershopper, says her quadruple A, size-11 foot makes buying shoes a source of frustration. "Instead I buy handbags. They're easy for me to find and I love them," she says.*

Another group of friends formed a Funny Feet Club after a chance remark tipped a conversation about each one's shoe size and the challenge it presents. One wears a 5½, two step out in 11s, three have triple or quad A skinny feet, and another is six feet tall and wears only size 10 flats. *"When we discover a shoe store with*

"Accessories can set a mood, send a signal, and entice."

wide size ranges or a sale with odd sizes available, we whip out our cell phones and dial up the Funny Feet Club," said Moira, an ophthalmologist.

The Internet opens a vast world of choices and instant gratification never before available, and the explosion of catalogs delivers a worldly smorgasbord of accessories into your life, regardless of where you live.

And life itself creates multiple options. You inherit stuff. Each year you celebrate personal events. You are seduced by novelties and new looks. You buy accessories while on a special vacation or when visiting an exotic place or store. As your income grows, so does yearning for "material" markers of success.

Rebecca had run out of space when she sent Judie an SOS for help. It wasn't clothing space that was the quandary, it was accessories. She had three drawers and two boxes full of real and costume jewelry. Another drawer overflowed with scarves of all sizes. Almost a hundred belts filled two belt rings, and another ring overflowed with long necklaces.

"I clean out my closet religiously every fashion season, but when it comes to accessories I just can't seem to part with anything," said Rebecca.

In addition to things she loves and has collected seriously, her drawers and boxes overflow with "could've beens," things she bought because she thought they would work with a particular outfit but they didn't. The vast choice muddles her thinking. Unlike clothes, most jewelry, bags, belts, and handbags don't shrink or get stains on them. That makes it harder to get rid of them. Rebecca had necklaces and bracelets that were ten or fifteen years old. When she looked closely at them she exclaimed, "These are from another lifetime. I would never wear them now. They are just not me."

Rebecca's hanging collection of belts, for example, revealed a veritable history of fashion trends back five or six years. Some of them made her laugh and confess she couldn't believe she ever wore them. And she rarely wore any of her beautiful scarves because she didn't think about them, stashed away in the lingerie chest. Out of sight, out of mind.

Pruning Rebecca's collection of accessories down to what she actually wore, and what she loved and hoped to wear, cleared her thinking on what outfits needed new accessories. We talked about trends this season that could update classic looks she already owned. Accessories become the exclamation points on these outfits.

It is easy to let this happen to you. In your twenties, everything is new; your life is filled with first-time experiences. In your thirties, you begin to refine your taste and it becomes more discriminating. In your forties, trends from your youth reappear, spiffed up for another go-round. Your friends start saying, "I remember the first time—," and twenty-year-old clothes are described as "vintage." By age fifty, your taste is secure. You travel, you observe; your eye is experienced, honed.

In each decade you take different approaches to the detail and accessory puzzle. Stay current with yourself. *Merril, a retired executive assistant, told us that during her career she acquired a beautiful collection of suits with shoes to match each and every outfit. Recently she donated all her suits to Dress for Success. So, where are the shoes, now that her suits are gone? She sheepishly admits, "I still have them on my closet shelf. I don't know what to wear them with now, but they are still in good condition so I'm saving them."*

Saving shoes by keeping them stowed in a box buries your options and their potential versatility as you move forward.

"I love the transforming power of accessories," says Bonnie, a specialty storeowner. "A white shirt and brown pants worn with an equestrian printed scarf, a beautiful leather belt, and riding boots speaks of old traditions, money, and a certain way of life. Put the same shirt and pants with western boots, a tooled belt with a big silver buckle, turquoise stones on a throat cord, and a western hat—and away you go to the barbecue."

The Challenge of Scarves

Scarves befuddle more women than all other accessories combined. Women complain about their inability to tie scarves—and once tied, how to make scarves stay put. Scarf companies produce brochures with indecipherable directions on how to tie them. At early seminars and speeches we dutifully demonstrated loops, bows, rectangles, and squares in various configurations. Then inspiration struck: *do women really need to know how to make a rose out of their scarf?* Keep it simple. Loop a longish rectangle around your neck and let the ends hang inside a jacket to add a bit of color, or simply loop the ends once and use a tiny safety pin as an anchor. Fold a large square into a triangle and use the old Girl Scout square knot method; right over left, then left over right. Tuck a square in your jacket pocket or tie it casually around your neck for a dash of color.

I feel that women are comforted by having clothes and accessories. I have every scarf I ever bought.

JUDITH KRANTZ, AUTHOR

Beautiful, colorful scarves reveal both your mood and your taste. Patterned scarves transform the simplest suit or dress into something distinctive. Choose swirls, floral, equestrian motifs, geometric or classic patterns to set a mood, your mood. Silk scarves are dressy, while knit scarves add panache to jackets and coats.

Be selective. Keep looking until a pattern calls to you or makes you think, "Yes, that's it, the perfect scarf for my outfit." You are entering a long-term relationship, as fine silk scarves, properly cared for, will last for years.

"Years ago, I saw the most beautiful scarf in a store window on Fifth Avenue. It was exceptional. Every major fall color was subtly worked into the pattern," said Elizabeth, an associate professor in English literature.

"I went inside, asked to see it, and then saw the price. It was really expensive, so expensive I considered framing it instead of wearing it as an accessory. I took a deep breath, pulled out my charge card, and bought it. That was seven years ago and I still absolutely love it. The silk is so beautiful and the colors go with about ten things in my closet. It was worth every penny."

Oversize triangle scarves make wonderful summer cover-ups when air-conditioning is too cool for your comfort. *Merri, a long, tall mood dresser, is ravishing each summer sporting her grandmother's fringed and embroidered piano shawl over colorful, simple tank dresses.* Be certain this type of scarf is in proportion to your figure.

JEWELRY TELLS THE WORLD ABOUT YOU

Your spirit, your romance, your reserve, your glamour, your whimsy, your no-nonsense attitude, and your life history swirl out from an aura you create of gold, pearls, glittering silver, twinkling diamonds (or make-believe sparklers), and the other stones you wear each day as jewelry.

Aura is an air, an attitude, the distinctive yet subtle quality of your character you project by your appearance. You know you've seen it. Stiff, erect, upright women emanating an aura of respectability. Striking women whose simplicity and style emanates elegance. Jewelry is the focal point of a woman's aura.

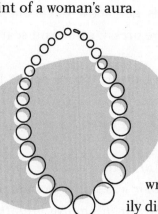

Jewelry expresses aspects of your personality, life, and beliefs: religion, alma mater, hobbies, marital status, economic status, birthday, taste level, and much more. Jewelry is emotional. It makes us feel desired, loved, or more attractive by lighting up our face or drawing attention to an elegant neck or slim wrist. It allows us to brag or be romantic. It readily discloses information to a perceptive observer.

As a single woman, what is the first thing you look for when you meet an interesting man? Number one checkpoint—is the guy wearing a wedding ring? Married men on the prowl *all* know the answer to that one. A light line where a wedding ring is supposed to be is a surefire giveaway.

Even early in life your taste in jewelry starts expressing your interests and who you are. As a youngster, most of your trinkets are about what your friends, peers, or the popular kids wear—pop star buttons, charms, or friendship bracelets. Your first precious jewelry is usually a locket or religious symbol on a tiny chain necklace. You store it in the velvet jewelry box it came in. Plastic watches, beads, coils, shells, fads, gewgaws, trinkets, and base metal baubles gain favor with you and then lose it.

In a special place you accumulate "good" jewelry, sentimental pieces from special friends, relatives, and parents such as dainty birthstone rings, I.D. bracelets, logo pins from organizations or clubs, pearls, and a good wristwatch. Talismans and charms may cast spells, making you feel lucky, powerful, blessed, or protected. You cherish certain mementos for the effect you believe they have on your life. Personal treasures arrive as life event markers. Each piece provokes a story or memories. Later you may receive fine jewelry: pearls, rings, diamond stud earrings, or other gems marking special celebrations. These may be unabashed "brag" pieces demonstrating wealth and success, your self-reward or self-worth being measured in carats.

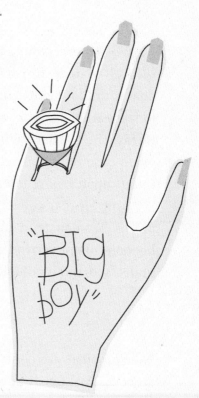

Ellen hurried in late for a monthly luncheon gathering of her birthday club. As she settled in, Elaine noticed a ring on Ellen's left hand. "Is that new? It's huge." "Oh, no," said Ellen with a wave of her hand, "I just don't wear 'Big Boy' very often, but I felt like taking him out today."

Okay. Let's talk. This Big Boy ring thing is out of hand. Blinding-size diamonds (if they *really* are diamonds) are an epidemic. Every village, suburb, and city meeting, drinking, and eating venue is filled with ladies of a certain age flashing Big Boy rings. What does this say about these women? Are they wealthy or just interested in giving that impression? Are they insecure and believe they need jewelry like this to be socially accepted or admired? Do you make judgments about a woman if she displays a Big Boy ring? We checked with our insider jewelry store connection, and she says cubic zirconium sells like crazy. Is it real? Only her jeweler or Home Shopping Network knows for sure.

> Jewelry isn't meant to make you look rich. It's meant to adorn you. And that is not the same.
>
> COCO CHANEL, DESIGNER

Women everywhere believe jewelry has to match: gold with gold, silver with silver, matte finish with matte finish. Pitch that thinking out the window, with that old maxim about no white shoes after Labor Day. Designers today readily mix gold and silver: look at David Yurman, Lagos, and John Hardy. The Cartier rolling ring is a classic mixing of gold and silver. Every piece of jewelry you select does not have to match everything else. Mix things up; it's more interesting.

Your all-real collection of finer jewelry becomes your basic jewelry pieces. Women tend to wear these pieces over and over because they become like a second skin. When you forget to wear a piece you feel undressed and incomplete, almost as if a part of you is missing.

SIZE AND SYMMETRY

Your physical size contributes to your sense of ease and pride in wearing an accessory. Small women occasionally carry off oversize or large pieces with great flair—but normally that is not the case. Neither does it mean petites must confine their choices to diminutive sizes. Beautiful and interestingly designed medium-size earrings are lovely on petite women. Conversely, small jewelry is lost on a full-figured woman; large pieces make her look less full in size. For example: a standard sixteen-inch necklace is an uncomfortable choker, or a tiny pin on a blazer doesn't "feel right." She will look balanced wearing a nineteen-inch necklace or a four-inch pin more in proportion to her size.

"It is important to consider scale and balance."

Experiment with a variety of jewelry sizes until you find your own most flattering proportion. Study your reflection in a full-length mirror. A woman with a long, slim neck gravitates to wearing necklaces. A beautiful pin on a jacket is a smashing attention getter. Placed high on a lapel or shoulder, a pin emphasizes the upper body horizontal line. A chunky pin embellished with beautiful stones also detracts from other areas you may wish to deemphasize.

Most fashion-smart women we meet have vast collections of earrings. Earrings are fun, glamorous, dramatic, and subtle and there's no problem with *fit.* You express your persona by sticking to simple studs (Classic/Romantic/Natural) or oversize hoops (Mood Dresser/Dramatic). Earrings add sparkle to your eyes, lift others' eyes to the face, and make most women feel "finished."

Review chapter 6, Proportion Politics, and consider how jewelry placement may accent your horizontal lines.

Tallying the Cost, Picking and Choosing

"Women want to wear real jewelry because of its value or sentiment," says Chris Gill, a former Saks Fifth Avenue accessory buyer and current merchandising executive for Tanner Designs. "Cost, however, restricts size. These real pieces are usually tiny, not impactful. So women turn to fashion jewelry."

There are exceptions. At the age of thirteen, Lori Lynne saw the old movie Gentlemen Prefer Blondes, *starring Marilyn Monroe and Jane Russell. It talked to her. "Marilyn played Lorelei Lee, which is almost my name, and when she sang "Diamonds Are a Girl's Best Friend" I knew she was telling me something. I must have watched that movie a dozen times. Marilyn was so glamorous. I decided I was going to collect diamonds. And I have." Lori Lynne has amassed a cache of diamond drops, studs, bracelets, wristwatches, and two dazzling necklaces. "My diamonds are mine alone and no one can take them away from me," she said. Her diamonds give her a sense of security and make her feel glamorous, ideas that resonated for Lori Lynne as a young teen and now.*

Costume jewelry is less expensive than "fine" jewelry. Most women collect costume jewelry: gold- and silver-toned earrings, bracelets and necklaces, plus items of faddish interest such as ethnic beads and chunky bracelets, pins, coral or amber strands, turquoise and silver. Fashion trends provoke you into buying an item, and weeks later you realize you never feel comfortable wearing it. It may be the wrong size for your body, or it may be outside your fashion persona.

Your fashion persona largely determines what type of jewelry you store. Trend trackers have boxes overflowing with "ins" and "outs" accumulated through seasons of rapidly changing styles. A Naturalist makes do with simple stud earrings and a strand of pearls. Miss Dramatic goes for impact. A Classic relies on familiar understated styles with proven effect. A professional woman, usually a Classic or a Modernist, is a special breed in that she wears jackets and therefore wears pins. Collecting pins becomes a form of persona expression, whether the pins are beautifully shaped and designed or playful. A Classic/Romantic might choose to wear a cameo or antique bar pin. Whimsical women wear holiday pins such as pumpkins, Christmas trees, hearts, or firecrackers.

Geography is destiny. Your birthplace and the places where you live influence your taste in jewelry. Women in the South, especially Florida, seek color and naturalism in their accessories. Shells, nuts, wooden beads, coral, and tropically influenced materials, whether carved or natural, are popular in casual jewelry. In the Southwest, Native American handicrafts define a whole genre of jewelry by artisanship and the use of silver and stones.

> "Experiment with a variety of sized jewelry until you find your own most flattering proportion."

Early in the 1990s designers created a new niche: costume jewelry touched up with gold or silver dips and semiprecious stones (their term) in distinctive styles, bearing stamps or signature motifs. This "designer jewelry," supported by elaborate advertising campaigns in glossy magazines, sells at hefty prices once reserved for precious metal and stone pieces. Among the fashion cognoscenti, identifying designer jewelry is a secret code detection game. Less modest designers sell bangles featuring their initials or last name. The brand has to be recognizable to have status, because then you and everyone else knows it. Consumers recognize this category of jewelry today as valuable and admired, despite a lack of value traditionally determined by carats or karats. It allows more women the opportunity to wear jewelry perceived as prestigious, without the price tag of fine gems and metals. And it fills a need, for jewelry today is aspiration as decoration. Jewelry is pure indulgence, a nonfunctional accessory.

Watches and Your Inner Self

Once upon a time, watches simply told you the time. Today watches are essentially variations of your inner self. A watch advertisement in a current *Vanity Fair* magazine has a single line of copy reading: "Who will you be today?" One watch serves as a billboard of your affluence, an "I'm worth it!" statement. Another watch is deemed casual, a diamond watch is dressy and sophisticated, and a Mickey Mouse watch is fun and flippant. The knockoff of a designer watch expresses your aspirations and good taste; and a watch equipped with special sport time mechanism says you are athletic. Like other accessories, we choose and select a watch to wear according to our mood, the occasion, or the season. Watches have become expressions of who we think we are and who we aspire to become.

SELF-EXPRESSION IN A HANDBAG

Handbags, pocketbooks, or purses, are miniature closets when it comes to diagnosing personality—and which word you use as a description is a tip-off to your age. Your grandmother Ada carried a pocketbook; your mom, Betty, carries a purse; and you carry a handbag. Messenger bags, mini-bags, baguette bags or totes—women own all kinds of shapes and sizes. The exterior adds or detracts from your personal aura. Inside, the valuables and odd things you carry around every day tell the tale of your inner psyche.

Emily swears her friend Jeanette "carries so much stuff in her gigantic bag she could do everything from delivering a baby to changing a tire with all the stuff in there."

What emotions do you stash in your handbag? Are you a "clutcher," hugging your bag close to your body with a death grip? Do you choose your handbag simply because you believe "it will go with everything," or "it will hold everything"? Must your bag burnish your status with famous initials or a logo, signaling social aspirations or self-worth?

Do you scoop up the latest fad bag, unaware of its shortcoming for your life? Be honest: when was the last time you really *looked* at your handbag and thought about what it says about you? Your persona dictates your style in acquiring and using handbags. Some women—Classics, Naturals, and perhaps Modernists, invest in one or two really fine bags. They keep the color neutral—black, navy, or beige—hardware discreet, and the shape simple. Other women such as Mood Dressers, Fashion Trackers, and Dramatics stock their shelves with trendy, diverse styles suitable for a variety of clothing and situations. An organized woman may depend on lots of zippers and compartments in her bag, while another woman may have a bag with two parts; one for her business endeavors, another for her family or spare time existence. You may slip from one philosophy to the other if your persona is a mix, such as Classic/Dramatic.

New York City street vendors have the instincts of Fashion Trackers as they display knockoff handbags so diligently copied from originals, it is difficult for most people to tell the difference between the genuine, pricey bags and the humbly priced copies. If you want to play the game, visit a fine store first and study styles, hardware, and the shape of authentic bags before snatching up a copy. Of late we hear of "handbag parties" in smaller cities, where a person presents and sells a variety of knockoff bags in a venue similar to old Tupperware parties. We think these inexpensive fakes are just fine for a fashion ego boost. Only you know for sure of its lineage, and six months later when the look is passé you aren't stuck with an expensive "out."

An oft-quoted adage says you can tell a lot about a woman by her handbag and shoes. We think the theory springs from England, a country with historical appreciation of fine footwear, and perhaps from Italy, a land noted for artisanship in leather. American women are often looked at askance in Europe because they underestimate the power of good shoes and a good handbag.

Late last summer, Barbara window-shopped Browns Boutiques on South Molton Street pedestrian mall, a stylish fashion destination in London. Her outfit was carefully chosen, yet as a nod to comfort she wore athletic shoes. A cocky English shop manager called out to her from his doorway, "Miss. You there, from the United States." She turned and said, "Yes?" "You are really quite an elegant lass, but those shoes ruin the whole impression," he said. While astonished by his rudeness, Barbara admitted his observation was correct.

Despite the importance you personally place on these accoutrements, finding shoes or a handbag that are functional, comfortable, and appropriate to your needs can be a trial. Strolling through a store, something catches your eye—a color, a shape, a pattern, and bingo, it is home in the closet. Women rarely think rationally about what a handbag will do for them.

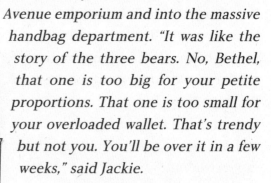

During a conference in New York, Bethel, venting frustration, cornered Jackie. "I cannot find the right handbag. I've been in and out of stores, circling counters for two days." Off they went to a famed Fifth Avenue emporium and into the massive handbag department. "It was like the story of the three bears. No, Bethel, that one is too big for your petite proportions. That one is too small for your overloaded wallet. That's trendy but not you. You'll be over it in a few weeks," said Jackie.

An hour later the duo was still at it, poking around inside bags, checking out side pockets, slots, zippers, and compartments. "This one is like a bucket; everything will fall to the bottom. Where will your cell phone go? Is there room for your wrap-around sunglasses, your cosmetic case?" prods the Dr. of Closetology. Another hour passes before they decide on the perfect bag. "I've got compartments for everything and a secure zipper slot in the center. It opens two ways, one for money, cards, and my checkbook, the other for my beauty goodies. It's the right size for my stature and I love it," said Bethel. This one won't sit on her closet shelf gathering dust.

Next time, *you* ask the questions. Pretend you are interviewing each bag for a position in your life. Think through your requirements and be certain that a new handbag, this vital extension of yourself, fills your needs and fits your body and style. Look in a full-length mirror and try on the shoulder strap. Where does the bag hit your body? Don't let it hang too low, empha-sizing your hips or derriere. What does the bag weigh? Is the lining well made of nylon or cotton? Is it heftier, cut of real leather?

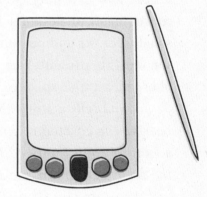

Use the same "interviewing" technique to select other accessory items you carry inside your bag. Wallets can be especially problemat-ical. You need to consider not only comfort but also security factors. After two pickpocket experiences, Judie carries one check in her wallet and credit cards in a separate case. Jackie has to have her complete checkbook as part of her wallet. Jennifer feels naked without her Palm Pilot. You may prefer a simple billfold with a zipper change pocket. Do ask yourself if all that stuff in your wallet such as your card stash is *really* nec-essary.

Your wallet, card case, and cell phone speak about you in a personal way, because they are on display each time you make a transaction. What you choose reflects both your taste and electronic savvy. Elegant, quality, coordinated pieces speak well of your organizational skills and indicate you've got your act together. Briefcases or portfolios are equally important, perhaps even more so if you do business with men. Men invest a lot of time and thought in purchasing their own business cases, and therefore notice what others select. Make yours sleek, elegant, and understated, leaving no doubt that they contain important papers for an important person.

An Initial Approach

Approach logo-laden handbags, wallets, checkbooks, and key cases with restraint, because prominently featured designer logos on clothes or accessories indicate you are image conscious or lack self-confidence. People today are very conscious of message tees, colors, and pictures of sports teams or designer logos, because they indicate the wearer's personal interests and personality, or are an indicator of an image that person wants to present. Wearing a logo or sports symbol repeatedly is a way of broadcasting a spirit or feeling that has priority in your mind.

Joanna tells a story about herself and her obsession with all things bearing the coveted LV initials. "Steve, my husband, and I were sitting in a lecture when I noticed he looked down at my friend's LV handbag on the floor, bent down, picked it up, and moved it over beside me. 'Excuse me! What are you doing?' said the woman, starting to rise. 'That is my wife's bag. I was just moving it out of your way.' Increasingly loud whispers erupted before Steve, embarrassed, sheepishly apologized. 'Sorry. I thought they all belonged to my wife.' "

As basic buying guidelines for handbags, keep in mind that crisp, geometric shapes in good leather (not split) are best with suits and tailored looks. Glossy black or reptile and skin patterns add an urban edge and a dash of formality. Slouchy, soft bags made of suede, canvas, nylon, fabric, or woven materials go with sporty, casual outfits. Preppy types traditionally favor a mix of canvas or nylon and rough leather trim for their casual bags.

For evening or special occasions, select a bag with a small to medium frame covered in very soft leather or fabric such as faille, jacquard patterns, or poly-satin, finished with distinctive hardware. Dressy evening events call for glittering beads and metallic materials or tapestry. Incidentally, it isn't necessary to spend a great deal of money on an evening bag. Discount stores and off-price retailers offer an array of evening bags at inexpensive prices.

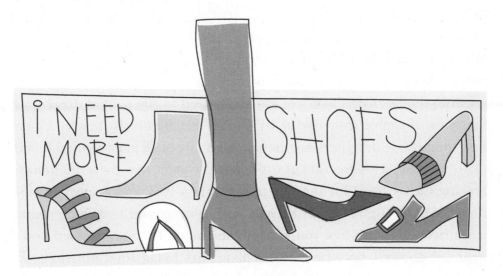

KICKING UP YOUR HEELS

I did not have three thousand pairs of shoes, I had one thousand and sixty.

IMELDA MARCOS

Cover up those bare midriffs (*so* very 2001–2002); the erotic hot spot today is feet. Flip open *Vanity Fair, Marie Claire, Harper's Bazaar,* or *Vogue* and there are shoes, baby, shoes! Strapped, wrapped, highlighted, sexy, shapely, sensual, and sky-high. Elegantly angled, deftly lighted, glossy, dramatic photographs present shoes in a seductive manner formerly reserved for high-powered sports cars.

Remember, please, most of this shoe hype emanates out of the Big Apple, New York City, where few people own cars or even have a driver's license. They walk a lot. When you walk, your shoes are noticed. And when you walk a lot you wear out shoes faster, thus creating a need to buy more shoes. In the rest of the world, women drive everywhere they go. If these women do walk very much, they wear athletic shoes or keep on hand a comfortable pair of shoes they know are good for walking.

> **"The best thing about shoes is telling your size doesn't mean a thing."**

Still, shoes, ankles, and feet are glamorized as the stuff of dreams, of fantasies, of sophisticated sexuality. High heels are overtly sexy and men love them. Shoe designers say they go for a mix of elegance with a touch of provocation. However, in our experience, women view them differently, seeking dressy heels for the way they create a look and a special emotional feeling. High heels make your walk alluring and body movements more riveting than when you wear driving mocs. But most women don't wear stiletto heels, because they just plain hurt. In fall 2002, stiletto heels on high fashion shoes soared to four or five inches. We do not wish to endorse any accessory that necessitates tolerating pain.

My sexuality and pleasure never had to do with my feet hurting.

CYBILL SHEPHERD, ACTOR

"I'm an absolute shoe fanatic," said Betty one August, as she trolled through a massive shoe department. "Last fall I fell hard for these killer stiletto-heeled boots with lacing up the back. They just reeked sex and fashion flash. I had to have them, even though they cost $540. My husband, Nicholas, did not believe me when I tried to explain them as an investment. *The heels are so high, wearing them is a test of endurance. I call them my pair of pain."*

Stiletto heels can also prove deadly to your business image. Short skirts and high heels à la *Ally McBeal* reruns are dumb ideas dictated by male television producers. In real life, such a getup makes males and females in any office wonder about the brainpower of the woman wearing such an inappropriate outfit.

 High-heeled, thin-strapped sandals have been known to drive some men to frenzies, but they're often men who want to tie you up.

CYNTHIA HEIMEL, AUTHOR OF *SEX TIPS FOR GIRLS*

Shoes have the power to enhance your body, your outfit, and the perception you wish to project. Shoes and boots also have an uncanny ability to make us feel taller, sexier, more solid and bold, or give our walk a bit of a swagger. Use them positively as a way of enhancing your overall image. Women's lives are complex and you need different types of shoes—some that are practical as well as some that give your ego a boost.

Lydia, a new client of Jackie's, says she heads straight to the shoe department of Saks, Bloomingdale's, and Macy's when she visits New York. "When I was a child I had polio, forcing me to wear ugly leg braces for years. My mother is a talented seamstress and she made me the most beautiful clothes, but all you could see were my ugly braces. When they finally came off, I got my first pair of black Mary Jane patent shoes. Even now, after all these years, I still remember the sheer joy of my first pair of pretty shoes," she said.

Foot problems—often caused by wearing toe-squeezing, overly high heels too often—plague countless women, creating limitations on the types of shoes they are able to wear. It may result in a loss of self-esteem.

Eve developed a serious foot problem requiring surgery, which resulted in her inability to wear anything but orthopedic shoes. "I feel so dowdy in everything I wear. It's taken the joy out of dressing up and buying clothes, because my shoes spoil everything," she said. A visit to a specialty shoe store offering a wider variety of styles helped, plus advice to wear pants and long skirts with trouser socks the same dark color as her shoes to minimize attracting attention to her ankle or foot.

One of the best things about shoes is that telling your size doesn't mean a thing. When a shoe sales associate asks your size, whether you answer 7, 9, or 10, you experience no embarrassing feelings of exposure. But emotional responses to shoes are a different matter. When your size is sold out in a shoe you are infatuated with, your emotions can help you rationalize buying a size that doesn't fit. *"I love it. I've got to have it."* Closets across the land are littered with shoes one size too small and too painful to wear.

BELTS: THE MIDDLE GROUND

Belts have a rich historical heritage dating back thousands of years, yet today, except for cyclical periods of fashion interest, belts tend to be selected for their functional use. Many women choose to simply bypass the waist entirely when they dress. Belt loops are removed from all new clothes without a passing thought. Others believe a belt adds color, texture, and finish to their appearance. A small percentage of women select belts with the same precision others reserve for pins or earrings, believing that a beautiful buckle is similar to a piece of jewelry and can be just as expressive of your personality. Full-figured women with hourglass silhouettes emphasize their waists with lovely belt buckles, creating an emphasis point under suit or dress jackets.

If you choose to wear belts, we advocate acquiring basic belts in good quality leather in a range of neutral colors such as black, navy, beige, and dark brown. You'll wear the black and brown belt for years, so if you can splurge, these two are the ones for your indulgence. If your budget allows, a glossy alligator or reptile skin belt delivers long-term use and a note of finesse. Embossed leather in similar patterns has the same fool-the-eye beauty as a knockoff designer bag. Buckles covered in leather are more subdued and less eye-catching than metal buckles, and don't detract from your other jewelry.

Keep your proportions in mind to gain the greatest benefit from belts. Belts the same color as your top visually lengthen the illusion of your torso. Belts the same color as your bottom pieces visually lengthen your legs.

Chain belts are another basic, because they help ease your proportions. A chain belt is worn slightly looser than a buckle belt, so you can adjust it to fall lower on your body. Presto, a woman with a short waist looks more in proportion, and a woman with a thicker waist suddenly looks slimmer. Simone, a friend with enviable continental flair, loves belts with a dropped chain loop attached to a leather belt or a chain belt with decorative coins on the loose end. Both visually detract from either wide hips or a large waist.

Periodically belts designed to be frivolous and flip, such as fringed, coin-bedecked, or jewel-encrusted collectibles, emerge briefly in favor. Belt connoisseurs love these moments in fashion, but alas, the waist has a disconcerting propensity to grow as one advances in years.

Even belt-cautious women fall for an occasional beautiful creation. Jackie still loves her sculptural silver 1980s Elsa Perretti belt buckle on a black leather cord. It serves as a dazzling piece of jewelry on her frequent all-black ensembles. Judie has a weakness for handcrafted, western silver concha belts in various forms, depending on them to spark up jeans and a basic shirt. This type of belt adds a special kind of dash when worn with suede jeans or a boot-length skirt.

GLASSES PROJECT ATTITUDE AND CHARISMA

Who knew, when Tom Cruise flipped his Ray Ban Wayfarers in *Risky Business* back in 1983, that a new accessory had just arrived? Within weeks, millions of Wayfarers sunglasses were sold in stores across the

United States, and they are still selling. And Cruise did it again by donning Ray Ban Aviators in *Top Gun.* The attitude conveyed by a pair of glasses exploded into a national obsession that is still rolling.

People use glasses to create a signature style, to hide their eyes and create a veil of privacy, or to forge impressions. While wireless glasses practically disappear on the face, tortoiseshell or dark frames connote seriousness and a bookish bent. Other frames convey perhaps a zany mood, or herald a season such as summer and surfing, or broadcast the panache of particular sport activities.

Fashion Trackers commit to an endless whirl (and hefty expense) trying to keep up with trends as styles in lenses, frames, and finishes race through "in" and "out" charts. Naturals often indulge in their glasses, favoring great outdoors styling, while Mood Dressers harvest vast collections. Joyce, a friend and jewelry designer, recently purchased a seven-foot-high commercial sunglass "spinner" display fixture to house her fanciful assortment of glasses.

The key to finding your persona in glasses is to patiently try on a bountiful variety. Try what's in *People* magazine this week, and then keep going until you find *you* in a frame. Face shape makes a difference. Generally round frames flatter angular features, and geometric, square, or angular shapes look best on round faces. An oval face seems to adapt to almost all types of frames.

ACCESSORIES ENTICE AND ADD FOCUS

In "Cinderella" as well as many other tales of courtship (think perfumed lace hankies), accessories have provoked action. Use them to your advantage. Begin by balancing your body overall with accessories, as most people see you as a whole when forming a first impression. Next use accessories to enhance your face and head, the second attention zone. On your midbody, use accessories to camouflage, emphasize, or detract. Use your hands and wrists to express, and your feet, shoes, or boots to intrigue.

Finding your personal accessories is a little like looking for love: first comes the search, then comes the excitement, and later, pure pleasure. You cast about looking for the perfect thing, and when you find it, you know.

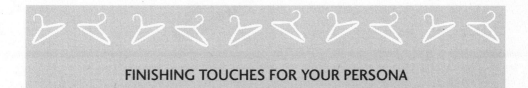

FINISHING TOUCHES FOR YOUR PERSONA

1. Dramatic—bold accessories: a pin, showcase necklace, unusual belt, fabulous boots
2. Modernist—a new variation on a classic, such as a sweater set updated with knit detail, lace or satin trim, or a different mix in lengths such as a hip-length cardigan paired with a waist-length turtleneck
3. Natural—pea coat, camel hair coat, all-weather trench, Polartec vest, a golden retriever, khaki walking shorts, real pearls
4. Mood Dresser—Slightly off-kilter mixes of colors, a wardrobe of different coat and jacket styles. Unusual belts. Sheer Boho/hippie tops. Long tiered skirts.
5. Romantic—ruffle trim on blouses, high band collars, subtle bands of inset lace, cameo pins, tiny estate jewelry pieces. Ankle-length hooded coat.
6. Trend Tracker—First with the color or accessory of the season. Latest boot, stiletto sandal, and advanced fashion coat. Faux fur muffler or hat.
7. Classic—beautiful trench coat, tweed topper jacket, beige flannel blazer, Newport-inspired summer sportswear

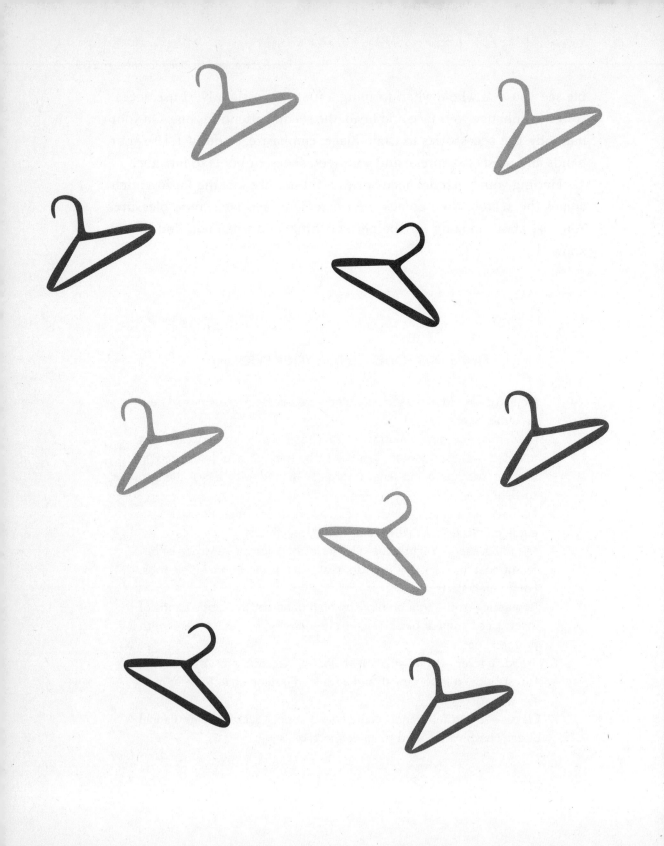

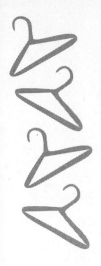

CHAPTER ELEVEN

TRAVELING: YOUR SUITCASE AS YOUR CLOSET

Is there anything as horrible as starting on a trip? Once you're off, that's all right, but the last moments are earthquake and convulsion, and the feeling that you are a snail being pulled off a rock.

ANNE MORROW LINDBERGH, AUTHOR

Karen has tennis elbow, but it is not from playing tennis. "I did it lifting my carry-on bag into the overhead bin once too often," she explains. "The orthopedic specialist said he had a cure, called 'check your luggage.' I hate to do that, because it takes so long to get in and out of airports." Judie sat down and talked Karen through her preparation process for each two- to three-day business trip. She discovered that Karen's "method" was to throw clothes in the suitcase for every possible event that might occur—dinner at a fancy restaurant, cold weather, warm weather, shorts, athletic shoes in case she wanted to jog.

Since we started this book, family and friends are accustomed to our asking strange and prying questions. So we did it again. We summoned four road warrior travelers for breakfast, hitting them with "How do you pack a suitcase?" Four different opinions, plus our two theories spilled forth.

Tanya is a roller devotee, Nancy compartmentalizes, Jane is an interlocker, and Paula is an obsessive chronological packer. *Break for a bit of explanation:* rollers and compartmentalize types are casual travelers fond of duffel bags and backpacks. You simply lay everything out flat, roll it up, and stack it in your bag, ending up with a suitcase resembling a cigarette

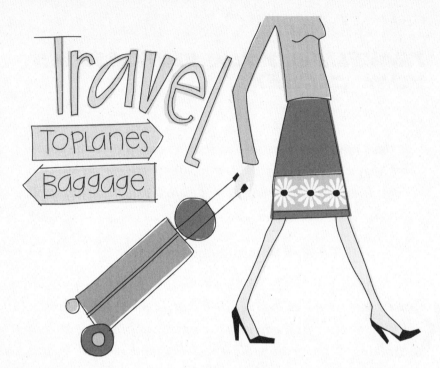

box. Compartment types put all tee shirts in one end, all pants in the other, and lingerie and sleep clothes in the middle, and other classifications stuffed in various side pockets. Interlockers master a complex system of interfolding their clothes into a kind of accordion. Chronological packers are superorganizers. They look at their trip schedule, put an outfit together for each day, then pack in layers with the first day's outfit on top.

Rolling creates a wrinkled mess for Judie, as she loves natural fabrics. Trying to interlock makes Jackie dizzy. We both use a variation of chronological planning. Most pieces of luggage accommodate a variety of packing methods. The advice we proffer was learned from trips covering thousands of miles and multiple cities both here and abroad, seasoned with pointers we wrung out of other women travelers and experts. Mainly we want to help you avoid mistakes we made back when we were young naifs and packed everything we owned.

THE MOST COMMON MISTAKES

The truth: bulging suitcases are monuments to indecision. You're in Chicago (Cleveland, New York, or maybe Miami), and once again you overpacked, unable to make up your mind. But you wanted to assure yourself that you would be ready for whatever wonderful occasions might come up. Who can blame you for that! Your suitcase is your on-the-road closet.

While we all try to develop our authentic selves, when you travel your luggage is not commodious enough to allow expression of the many experimental aspects of your personality. Packing requires discipline and objectivity.

Knowing how to pack for any type of trip ought to be enshrined as the eighth Habit of Highly Effective People, if best-selling author Stephen R. Covey will allow us to suggest an addition to his best-selling book.

Like Karen, the gal with tennis elbow, you may have so many "What if" ideas while packing that you can't focus on what *will* happen during upcoming travels. Packing this way is overcompensating for the sense of insecurity you feel about your trip. But there are other packing pitfalls. Do any of the following seem familiar?

Sheila, a business travel novice, found herself in a snowstorm in Indianapolis and the warmest thing in her suitcase was a wool blazer. Why? "I didn't think it would still be cold here," she said as her boss gallantly whipped off his coat and draped it over her shoulders. She's now a fan of travel forecasts on The Weather Channel.

The *"we're not in Kansas anymore, Toto"* syndrome affects women who want to dress in tune with their destination, and this can provide more insecurities than jet lag. Maggie, a normally tuned-in, hip kind of young woman, stepped out on Fifth Avenue in New York one summer day and started people-watching for trends. Soon she noticed no one was wearing summery white shoes but her. The farther she walked, the bigger and more out of place she felt her feet become. "I had to go back to the hotel and change, because I felt like Minnie Mouse," she said.

In big cities and other countries, dress codes differ, and you need acute radar to pick up appearance signals. Women in New York love to wear black. In Los Angeles, they opt for chic neutrals or brighter colors. You would be as out of place wearing pastels in Chicago as all black in Palm Beach. Globe-hoppers jetting to Europe or Scandinavia leave white jogging shoes and shorts at home. They mark you as an American tourist and are considered tacky. Check ahead and dress appropriately.

Flushed with excitement, Dramatic persona Lizbeth looks upon each journey as an *adventure of self-expression.* She spends hours sorting through her closet, shopping in stores, changing blouses, shoes, and

"Bulging suitcases are monuments to indecision."

accessories for her outfits—even though Lizbeth takes twenty to twenty-four trips a year. "People expect me to look like a trendsetter, so I always overpack and am exhausted by the time I take off," she moans. Lizbeth suffers from an affliction we call competitive dressing. Like a casting director, she presents herself as a trendsetter as a means of individuating her personality and impressing other people. Then, lacking a costume designer or wardrobe stylist, Lizbeth goes hunting for outfits she feels suit a trendsetter. No wonder she is exhausted.

Traveling, whether for business or pleasure, is stressful, challenging, and tiring. Navigating airports, keeping on schedule for connecting flights, standing in long lines, and going through multiple security searches take a toll. Then there is the specter of lost luggage, a fear serious enough to intimidate seasoned jet-setters.

A MASTER PLAN

The savviest traveling women we meet know that when you live out of your suitcase, you must condense your fashion persona, and replace waffling guesses about climate and locale with knowledge-based facts.

Face it: for most business or pleasure trips, you can narrow your needs by preplanning and researching. Be spartan. Zero in on the weather at your destination; visit city and country Web sites for local knowledge. Even the smallest cities and towns today have Web sites, and you can get a sense of what the area is about by scanning them. Travel sites such as Fodors.com are brimming with information. Scan newspaper travel sections for weather. Make a practice of saving travel stories on cities or countries you plan to visit. Call it your fun file. Better yet, talk to someone who recently visited where you are going. Business travel atlases include drawings of major airports with tips on mass transit and costs. Study these, and turn that knowledge into confidence. Confidence is always more impressive than perfect makeup or a brand-new suit.

We hear you protesting: "It takes too much time." What about all the time you spend rustling through your closet and waffling on what you think you may need for a trip? Add up the time you spent shopping for clothes you think you want, may not be able to afford, and might not even wear. All that stuff you pack eats up time: packing, unpacking, hanging it in hotel closets and stashing it in bureaus, pressing, then packing again, lugging it to the airport, getting home, and unpacking again. The next day you have to launder it or take it to the dry cleaners; even the things you didn't wear have to be pressed again. That all adds up to a lot of your time.

Trips fall into standard categories such as business, weekend escapes, weeklong vacations, grand tours in the United States or foreign countries, and visits to relatives. Travel experts say 65 percent of all trips are eight days or less. Tune your thinking and planning into categories, as each type of trip calls for a different approach to dressing.

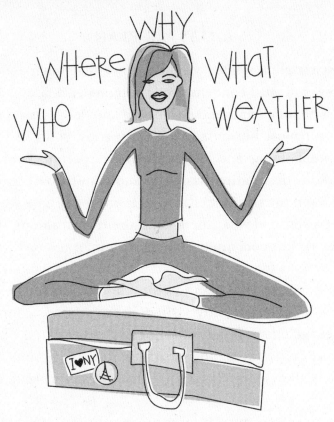

THE FIVE *WS* OF SUITCASE SIMPLIFICATION

1. *Who* is going on this trip? Are you responsible for planning and packing for you, your partner, or more family members? Who you are traveling with may influence how formally or informally you feel you can dress.

2. *Where* are you going and how many days will you be gone?

3. *Why* are you going? Is it a business trip, weekend getaway, family vacation, or a romantic escape?

4. *What* activities will you be doing? Do these activities involve special clothing you need to pack?

5. *Weather* is a key issue. Will you be traveling to one or several destinations? What is the weather there going to be?

DO YOUR WEIGHT LIFTING AT THE GYM

One rule doesn't change. *Travel with as little as possible.* Redcaps, bell-men, luggage handlers, porters, and stewards are vanishing species. If you can't lift your luggage yourself, you've packed too much. One bag checked and/or one carry-on is your desired max.

Being a road warrior businessperson and gold medallion frequent flyer sounds glamorous until reality hits on a stormy afternoon when you dash from your rental car across the parking lot (unassisted), stand under a leaky bus pavilion, wrestle your luggage onto the van, ride to a terminal, wrestle your suitcase off, and struggle across oncoming traffic and into the terminal, only to face an endless line of people, soaked like you, all waiting to check in.

Trust us. You want to be able to lift your own luggage—even for that long-awaited grand tour of Europe that's finally become a reality. In Europe, traveling by rail rules. Someone (read you) has to get your bags on and off trains, buses, or the Chunnel, in and out of those rustic bed-and-breakfasts, through airports and customs. Pensions in Italy can be wonderful, but for some reason most come with rooms on the third or fourth floor, accessible only by ancient winding staircases.

"Traveling for business or pleasure creates a mix of emotions."

You want to look wonderful. You want to be impressive. You want to be appropriately dressed. You also want to be smart.

STARTING WITH THE BASICS

In an unscientific poll of traveling women, we discovered each owns at least two pieces of wheeled luggage. The first is a typical carry-on, multi-zipper bag designed to fit under the seat in front of you or in the overhead bin. The second piece is large, capable of holding fifty to seventy pounds, with a sturdy pull handle. Rules may vary, so check with airlines for exact measurement and weight details, especially if you are traveling to foreign countries.

"You want good luggage but I always suggest avoiding status luggage, the kind with designer logos all over it," says travel agent Diane Larson. *"It screams 'steal me, I'm full of expensive stuff.' And porters expect double their usual tip for handling it."*

Instead of a stiff briefcase, most of these women love the flexibility of a leather or heavy vinyl tote bag large enough to hold a slim laptop, cell phone, makeup case, travel documents, survival gear (must-haves in case your luggage goes astray), and personal essentials such as books, notepads, etc. You must also be able to slip your handbag inside this tote during boarding, as most airlines allow only two carry-on pieces.

One favorite tote, twelve to fourteen inches high by sixteen inches wide, is divided into several sections with one zippering shut for security, and several side pockets inside as well as one flapped side pocket outside. The flapped pocket is handy for travel documents, tip money, directions, a comb, and lipstick. Strong, flat, one-inch-wide straps slip easily over your shoulder.

Start every trip with an extensive written itinerary. If you are traveling with someone else—your husband, a business colleague, or a friend—share this itinerary with them to avoid slipups.

Jocelyn was excited about her first trip to Las Vegas with her husband. As always, they each packed for themselves. The second night, as Jocelyn prepared to dress for a poolside luau, she noticed Neal dressing in a business suit. Mustering up diplomacy she inquired, "Did you bring something islandlike for tonight?" His face went blank. He thought it was an all-business trip. Later they realized they had not discussed the itinerary during their hectic days preparing to get away.

On your itinerary, plan day by day using a vertical format. Fill in your anticipated appointments or activities by approximate hour or day segments, including travel, lunch plans, and evening meetings or restaurant destinations. Note beside each activity what you will wear.

For example, on initial airplane travel days, we always recommend wearing a pantsuit with a blouse or shirt you want to wear but know will wrinkle if you pack it. A black pantsuit with a high Lycra content is a perfect choice, as you can easily dress it up, dress it down, or wear the pieces separately. Lycra gives your pantsuit stretch ability so it is comfortable, retains its shape, and is virtually wrinkle free. Wear your heaviest shoes and carry your coat or outer jacket. On a three-day trip you could wear the same pantsuit home, teamed with a different bright-colored knit top.

Long hours on flights cross-country or abroad call for soft dressing, such as sweater sets with easy fitting pants, or matched knit sets such as a tunic and slim pants. Judie tells her daughters to find something comfortable as pajamas. You want to look well turned out yet be comfortable. If you have to go directly to a meeting or dinner on arrival, wear your suit to the airport, but tuck casual pants and a top in your briefcase or in a zipper compartment of your carry-on bag. After the plane is in the air, change into your comfy clothes, and lay your good outfit flat in the overhead bin. Before landing at your destination, change back into your suit.

As you fill in your itinerary and clothing choices, think versatility. For a dressy dinner, that travel pantsuit could be teamed with a shimmering satin blouse or glittery top and sexy, high-heeled sandals.

When you finish your trip list, count up the approximate number of outfits you anticipate needing, and immediately try to eliminate or combine a few choices. A traveler's rule of thumb is to calculate what you think you need to take, then cut it by half. *A confession: we've never been able to do that, but it gives you something to shoot for!*

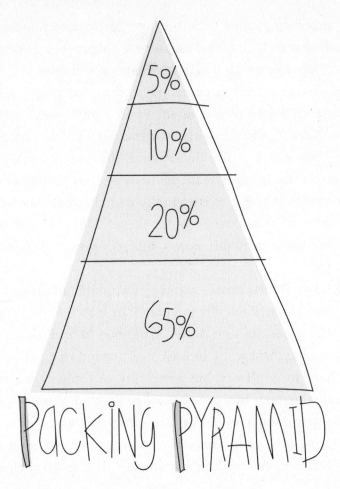

A PACKING PYRAMID

Another way to focus on actual travel needs is to form a packing pyramid. First you decide the classification of clothing you need the most. This forms the bottom of your pyramid. For example, on a business trip your largest classification will be business attire. Then add evening attire such as dining out, theater, concerts, or club hopping; casual or workout wear; and any special event, which might be a semicostume night, such as a roundup barbecue at a convention or an awards banquet. The pyramid would look like this for a five-day business trip with one day on your own:

Special event	5%	Silk shantung dress and jacket
Evening	10%	Jersey separates, black jeans, sparkle tee, silk shirt
Casual (include in-room loafing and something to wear when you get room service)	20%	Knit pants, tees, black jeans, hooded sweater jacket
Business	65%	Black pantsuit, silk shell, coral knit tee, beige jacket, print silk skirt and top, cream-colored jacket, pants, and jersey shell top

The pyramid forces you to crystallize your thinking on actual needs—business attire—versus a bouquet of options you might be tempted to pack for evening, which you quickly see account for only 10 percent of your activities.

Using this outline, list each outfit planned, then note shoes, accessories, special lingerie or hosiery, and jewelry. You could easily eliminate the jersey separates (skirt, pant, shell, and jacket) and utilize your business pieces for evening.

In this next example, it's vacation time and you plan to go on a ten-day singles cruise. Check the itinerary from the cruise line and circle activities that attract your interest. You

PACKING FOR A WEDDING, GRADUATION, OR CHRISTENING

For important events, you'll need a more structured bag such as a carry-on size wheelie or a hang-up garment bag that meets security restrictions. To avoid lost luggage slipups, keep the bag with you on the plane. We like wheelies equipped with a separate, built in, fold-up hanger compartment. Create your packing list from your itinerary of events. Be sure to ship or mail any gifts, as airlines no longer allow wrapped packages as carry-ons.

quickly realize casual clothes will be the norm 70 percent of the trip, both in ports and on deck. For three special nights, plus the last-night captain's party, you want cocktail club clothes, adding up to about 15 percent. Swimwear, workout gear, and sleepwear fills out the balance 10 percent. Presto, you've got your cruise packing pyramid!

DO A DRESS REHEARSAL

Stage a dress rehearsal prior to packing. Take each outfit and lay it out on your bed, complete with lingerie, shoes, handbags, jewelry, belts, and scarves. Make a final check for missing buttons, loose hooks, or other maladies. This way, you see your entire trip clothes package. You will discover that "I could leave this behind and wear that with that."

"Stage a dress rehearsal prior to packing."

After working out these "capsule" plans for several business trips it becomes easier to pack, because you understand exactly what goes with what for similar future trips. You learn which pieces really work well for you and can focus on buying similar replacement pieces when the need arises.

For vacations, this itinerary plan is priceless. Pack a copy in the suitcase. It saves you time whenever you dress, as you have predetermined what you want to wear and what goes with what. We suggest you pack categories together in layers. Using the example above, you would group business wear, casual, evening, and special event. On vacations you would want to group jeans and casual bottoms with knit tops and tees, to remind yourself of the mixing and matching possibilities.

Avoid travel goofs by doing dress rehearsals. Libby, an *über*-stressed junior executive, used to claim she didn't have time for them until essentials came up missing in action on two back-to-back trips—the skirt to her "presentation" suit on the first trip and a strapless bra to wear with her banquet ensemble on the second. Every well-traveled woman has a story like that to tell, including designer Vera Wang, who admits her most famous fashion faux pas was wearing two different colored pumps to a White House luncheon. (*Vogue,* April 2002).

WHAT GOES WHERE?

Most packing experts suggest putting handbags and lumpy grooming aids such as hair dryers and barrel-style hairbrushes in first, on the bottom of your suitcase. Save space and weight by calling ahead to your hotel and checking if hair dryers are provided in your room. The next layer is lingerie, hosiery, sleepwear, and soft casual wear, then tissue- and plastic-wrapped pants, tops, blouses, and dresses. Judie is a fan of packing with plastic dry cleaner bags and zipper storage bags. "I put a plastic bag over a blouse on a hanger, then put a jacket over that, and another plastic bag over that. Each dress and skirt gets its own plastic bag. I layer all my pants on top of each other, put tissue in the middle, then fold them all once on each other. Lotions, scarves, and hosiery all are stashed in zipper bags. It keeps everything protected and together." Prior to trips, put dry cleaner bags into an empty suitcase so they are there when you pack.

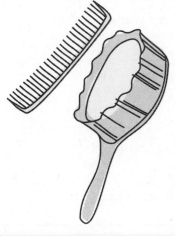

Jackie flips the procedure. She packs bulkier pieces such as jackets on the bottom, and then creates layers of sweaters, skirts, pants, blouses, tees, and camisoles, keeping each classification together. Sweaters or fragile items that may snag are zipped into plastic bags as the top layer. Sleepwear and lingerie go in a mesh compartment in the top of her bag. Accessories go into sandwich zip bags and are tucked into open spaces. She covers all her clothes with a plastic sweater bag, saving shoes and her cosmetic bag for last on top.

A few caveats: never pack shoes or handbags empty. Stuff them with trouser socks, thongs, boxer shorts, or other small items. The toes of your pumps are great for stowing items wrapped in tissue or inside a plastic zip bag. Separate matching shoes, as they are easier to position.

"Survival gear" goes into your tote or carry-on bag, if you check luggage. This smoothes the way somewhat if your luggage goes to Omaha while you are going to Los Angeles. Pack prescription drugs in their original containers, makeup basics, and small, disposable containers of toiletries, your jewelry, a bra and panties, hosiery, a knit top, and any medications you require. We also throw in a few energy bars to stave off starvation on food-free flights or middle-of-the-night arrivals.

Brooks and Pat, two seasoned travelers, said their "survival gear" eased the stress when their luggage was lost for three days en route to a cruise. "It helped people get to know us, because when you wear the same outfits for three days, people tend to remember who you are," she said.

SURVIVAL GEAR OPTIONS—
THINGS YOU MAY WANT TO PACK

1. A few favorite books and/or magazines to read en route or during airport layovers.
2. Journals or index cards to jot notes or information on people you meet.

3. An ample supply of standard business cards, plus E-mail-only business cards.

4. A supply of 8½-by-11-inch envelopes to mail home used guidebooks, souvenirs, and books you've read and want to keep in your library.

5. Extra contact lenses or reading glasses.

6. A small package of tissues. Keep a couple in your pocket at all times.

COLOR PLANS

The easiest way to confine your clothing choices is to select no more than three colors. Use one basic color for bottoms, and add variety with switchable tops in matching solids, contrasting stripes, and prints.

Sample Packing Capsule for a Four-to-Five-Day Business Trip

Black jacket, skirt, and pants

One pair of black-and-white tweed or houndstooth check pants

Tops: One black knit top, one black-and-white-striped knit top, one red sweater set, one print shirt or silk blouse

Black pant shoes, black pumps, black daytime bag, black evening bag, plus accessories

Total: four-to-five outfits

1. Black jacket, skirt, and silk blouse
2. Black jacket, striped knit top, and black pants
3. Red sweater set, tweed or check pants
4. Black jacket, black knit top, tweed or check pants
5. Red sweater set, black skirt

Capsule for Three-to-Four-Day Business Trip

Gray pants and jacket

Gray, black, and red geometric print skirt and blouse

Coral shell top

Black silk shirt or knit top

Red sweater set

Black pant shoes, red pumps, black daytime bag, black evening
  bag, accessories

Total: four outfits

1. Gray pants, jacket, coral top

2. Print blouse, skirt, and gray jacket

3. Red sweater set and print skirt

4. Gray jacket, pants, black blouse

PIVOTAL PIECES ADD VERSATILITY

Pivotal pieces are items that travel well and offer versatility. They become
your trusted wardrobe friends, always there for any occasion.

1. A "stand alone" jacket. This jacket is not attached to a particular skirt, pant, or suit. It gives you a pulled-together look
   and can be worn with everything from a wool trouser to jeans.
   Some candidates: a cream blazer in baby corduroy or raw silk,
   a black leather jacket, a jean jacket, and in the Sunbelt, a
   short-sleeve white jacket to pop over tees and pants or skirts.

2. A dressy something. This could be a jacket, skirt, or top in a
   dressy fabric, or one embellished with beads, sequins, or
   appliqués. It could be a collectible "art to wear" find or a

hip, sparkly tee shirt with Op or nostalgic art. It gives punch to your wardrobe and fills the bill if you head out for clubbing at the last minute.

3. A wrap. Legions of women swear by their scarves, shawls, and wraps. These oversize scarves are handy to add color, coverage, or warmth on a chilly evening. Sun worshipers love them because you can tie it on as a skirt, as a quick strapless or halter sundress, and in a pinch, use it as a beach blanket.

4. A casual pant. Our favorites are black jeans, khakis, or an easy knit pant. After a day of traveling and working, you want something comfortable to change into. Team the pants with your favorite tee, sweatshirt, or tunic for in-room lounging, or to be presentable when room service arrives, or wear it with one of your blouses for a spiffy casual look for dinner or a movie.

5. A simple jersey or crinkle cotton and Lycra dress. A simple little black dress can do wonders to extend your travel wardrobe. You can dress it up with heels, a shawl, and pearl earrings, or wear it by day with sandals, sunglasses, and a straw bag. There is a great selection at www.Travelsmith.com.

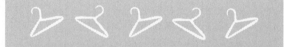

PACKING FOR A WEEKEND GETAWAY

Choose an eighteen- to twenty-three-inch-wide duffel or similar size soft bag, especially if you're traveling by car. Show style in your choice of bag. Opt for a bright color, stripes, contrasting handles or straps. Cotton canvas is great on a boat or in a car, as it allows you to fit more pieces of luggage in a small space. Heavy-duty canvas or vinyl duffels are a safer bet if you must check your bag. Look for a bag with a wide opening top or a U-zipper that allows you to flip out one side.

A Typical Summer Weekend Packing List
Color coordinate one skirt, one pair of pants, one pair of shorts, two tops, a sweater or light jacket (depending on activities and locale). Then toss in a swimsuit, two pairs of shoes, toiletries, sleepwear, and underwear.

PACKING TIPS

Do you have three cities in three days on your itinerary, with varying temperatures? Layer up and layer down using tees, sweaters, and jackets.

Wise women never pack new shoes on a trip.

If you are a member of a frequent flyer club, take your membership card so you can board planes first, when overhead bins are still empty.

Buy and pack a small portable clothes steamer if you can't stand wrinkles. Sometimes hanging your clothes in the bathroom with the shower blasting hot water just doesn't get the job done.

Two travelers said they pack old clothes or old lingerie. During the trip they simply throw away each item after they've worn it, freeing up space in their suitcases for souvenirs. It's a thought.

Consider packing a compact, folding bag with a zipper in your luggage, so if you shop during your trip, you'll have a way to get souvenirs and goodies home.

A frequent traveler to Italy starts saving the ends (about the last quarter) of bathroom tissue rolls prior to trips to Tuscany. She lines the bottom of her suitcase with them, protecting gifts she is taking back to relatives—and

PACKING FOR A
TEN-DAY TO TWO-WEEK TRIP
Start with one large wheelie bag or two smaller, different-size bags. The smaller bag, perhaps a tote, should be able to loop over the handle of the larger one. Be sure you can handle and lift the bags yourself. A canvas tote is handier on a fun trip, as it can double as a beach bag, book bag, picnic carrier, or fresh market shopping bag.

Packing list
One dress, one skirt, three pants, and five tops: one to coordinate with the skirt, four to mix and match with pants. A sweatshirt, two lightweight sweaters, or a sweater set, jacket, or raincoat (depending on destination), four pairs of shoes, swimsuit and cover-up, underwear, sleepwear, and toiletries.

while in her homeland, she has soft tissue for herself. It's a good idea when traveling to a lot of foreign countries!

It's okay to stash your capsule wardrobe in the back of the closet for a while after you return from a lengthy trip. Like maternity clothes, many women don't want to see these clothes again for a long time.

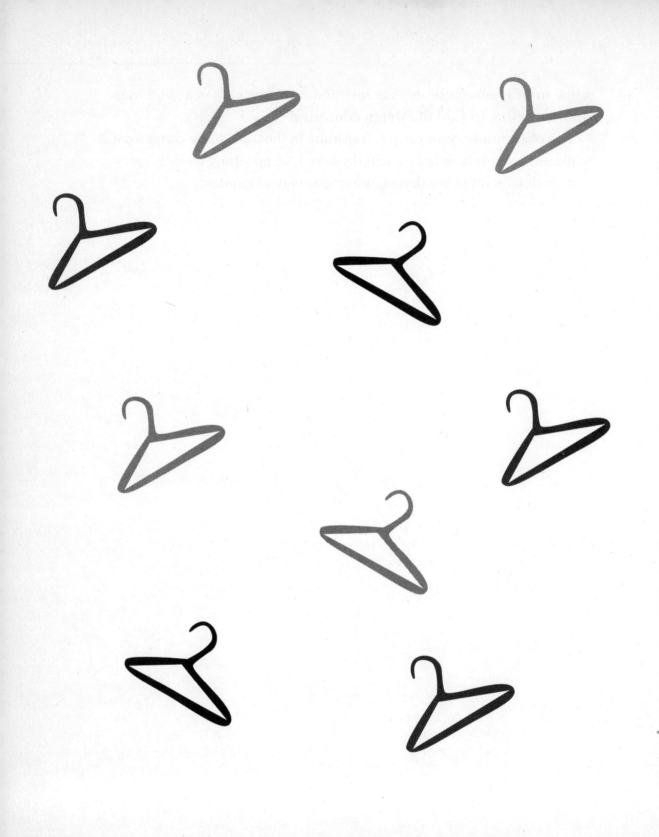

FIFTY BONUS HOT TIPS

INSIDER SECRETS YOU NEED TO KNOW

- Wednesday or Thursday nights are great nights to stop by stores, as sales personnel are often putting out fresh markdowns and sale items for weekend specials. Don't hesitate to ask if something you are interested in buying will be going on sale soon.

- Try on items from more expensive brands or collections than your usual budget can handle. This enables you to know how they fit, and you'll be ready to buy quickly from catalog sales or end-of-the-season sales when things get marked down 50 or 75 percent.

- Check to see whether your favorite stores offer charge accounts or "frequent shopper" cards. Find out what perks they might offer, from monthly discount certificates to notices of private sales for special customers only. Several women's chains send out monthly folders with 20 percent discount coupons. One company sends out a "happy birthday coupon," good for a 50 percent discount on one item to registered members.

- When you need to buy new bras, call your favorite store and make an appointment to be fitted. Many stores now offer this service, and it saves you money and time by avoiding fit mistakes.

- Take inventory of your bras and be certain you have all the styles you need. Many women don't. You should have smooth finish cups to wear with knits, sport bras for workouts or tennis, wide-set-strap versions for scooped necklines, and strap-less or low-cut bras to wear with bare summer clothes and special-occasion outfits. And every woman needs an indulgent, sexy, lacy bra.

- Shopping for jeans is a major challenge. One popular women's magazine reports that the average woman has to try on thirty-two styles to find the right one for her body! Believe it or not, it's worth it to make time to do this. Whether your jeans fit well or poorly, you will wear them a lot. If they fit your body well, you'll feel great—not grubby—every time you put them on. (We also recommend trying on five different pairs of the one style you select. Frequently, each pair differs slightly in fit and length.)

- Look for 5 to 6 percent Lycra in pantsuits, jackets, skirts, and pants. It helps keep fabrics from wrinkling, is comfortable, and enhances fit.

- Sheer and illusion-type fabrics are great for revealing while concealing. A bare back or arms veiled with sheer net lets you dare to wear barer looks at any age. This is one of Sophia Loren's greatest fashion tricks.

- Long opera-length bead necklaces or pendent necklaces falling below your bustline create a vertical, slimming line.

- A long vertical stole or shawl draped over one shoulder makes you instantly look taller. Drape it around your neck, with the ends romantically trailing down your back, to camouflage a neck you wish looked better.

- Black does not look summery or casual. Opt instead for wearing one bright color top to toe, a snazzy print pant, or a zingy citrus-colored top over dark, neutral pants or walking shorts.

- Splurge on a wonderful coat you really love in a beautiful, quality fabric. It's one of the items you wear the most, and you want it to last.

- Never buy a long winter coat in a bright color. You'll be sick of looking at it before the season is half over. Instead go for a colorful short coat or a bright jacket that works both for daytime and sport.

- If you live in a Sunbelt state, train yourself to shop the resort collections, which arrive in stores just before Christmas and through January. Down south, hot weather keeps you in lightweight clothes more than six months. Buying from resort collections gives you a longer time to wear your new looks.

- Give yourself a browsing shopping day at the beginning of each new fashion season. Use it to analyze trendy items, new colors, and silhouettes. Try on new styles to see if they are for you.

- When you go on a serious shopping mission, dress for action. Choose easy-to-slip-off clothes and shoes and minimal jewelry, and tuck your favorite support panty hose in a tote so you'll know "for sure" how a slim skirt or dress will really fit.

- Fragrance is part of your wardrobe too. It should be shorthand for an aspect of your personality. The next time you're in your favorite department store, spend a pleasant half an hour trying on perfumes. Note the names (Escape, Happy, Romance, Joy, Beautiful, Pleasures) and ask yourself whether the lingering scents seem to suit you and speak to who you are.

- In catalogs, be aware that clothing is usually not form-fitting. This ploy cuts down on returns for the catalog company. Read descriptions for indicators such as "slim fit," "low-rise waist," or "boxy cut," and carefully check size charts in the middle of catalogs for measurements.

- If a shirt or pants looks good in a new or unfamiliar catalog, order one for a "try on." If you like the fabric and the way it fits, order more in other colors, then buy replacements for next year from their end-of-the-season clearance.

- Capri pants are great for summer, and everyone has a crop spot on their calf that is most flattering. Study your look in a full-length mirror and find your sweet spot.

- Do not shop for flat-front skinny pants on a Monday, unless you spent the weekend at a spa.

- The quickest way to visually elongate your silhouette is to wear a bright or light-colored jacket over dark or neutral-colored separates.

- One-shouldered tops, wrap dresses, and sarong-style skirts are great fool-the-eye for slimming silhouettes. The eye follows the line of the clothes.

- Finding the right skirt length for you and sticking with it saves time when putting outfits together. Different skirt lengths require different shoes, jacket lengths, and stockings.

- Stripes create magic proportion illusions. A bold wide stripe across the bust makes your bust look larger. A wide stripe at the bottom of a tunic top emphasizes the hips. Stripes starting at the shoulder and diminishing in width above the waist make your waist appear smaller. Vertical stripes up the side of your pants add length to your legs.

- Develop a relationship with a nearby consignment store, so you will have a place to sell your "mistakes" and older styles.

- Change buttons on your clothing to update them, or to change a piece from corporate to dress. Remember that good buttons make clothes look more expensive.

- Buy wardrobe additions carefully. Whether it is a color that makes you look fabulous or a flattering silhouette, everything you buy should be a projection of who you are.

- Do a walking tour through major stores to study new arrivals and what is featured. You will notice repeats of the same dress or sportswear groups. Avoid buying these, to avoid running into women dressed just like you.

- Indulge yourself by using odd bits of frequent flyer mileage to purchase items. Many national chains and specialty stores participate in these programs.

- A store specialist may best supply your special need. Call and inquire about personal shoppers, fitting specialists, and other knowledgeable individuals. They can save you time and solve your problem.

- At least once a month, take time to shop in your closet. We've discovered many new looks and we love using this method.

- Look in the Yellow Pages of your phone books under Clothing Manufacturers and Catalogs. Call and inquire if they have a factory outlet or seasonal sales. Many do, and savings are significant.

- Always ask out-of-town friends for their favorite stores in their hometown. Native knowledge leads to outstanding and one-of-a-kind shopping destinations.

- When seasons change or your hair color changes, your makeup must change to match your new color tones.

- Irene, our fragrance guru, suggests each woman select four fragrances: (1) for work that is "you" but not strong, (2) a sexy, musky scent for dates and big nights on the town, (3) a light, fresh fragrance for outdoors activities, and (4) an impulsive scent that is your favorite.

- Before taking a trip by car, check in the travel section of your bookstore for "outlet directories." You will uncover great shopping finds. At your destination, check in at the travel/local section of a bookstore there for such directories that are not sold nationally.

- When buying and trying on clothes, pay attention to fabric. Be aware of how it feels on your body, so you won't get it home and suddenly discover it is scratchy. Observe how the fabric falls over your body, and be sure it meets your standards.

- On quick travel trips it is safer to confine your shopping to accessories, as they are less of a hassle to mail back if you get home and decide you don't love them or they don't fit. And with accessories, you can always give them to someone else.

- Keep a list of all of your charge account numbers and company phone numbers in a secure place. If your wallet or handbag is stolen, you can quickly call and report the theft. Also file a police report and get a case number. The latter is especially important when traveling by airline, as the report is a substitute for your photo I.D., authenticates the theft for credit bureaus, and may prevent you from being charged for a replacement driver's license.

- Keep a list of the phone numbers of your favorite shopping destinations in your wallet, calendar, or Palm Pilot. Include a sales associate's name. When you see an ad in the paper or article in a store catalog, you can quickly call your person to hold that item, check if it is in stock, or charge and send it to you. This can be a great time-saver.

- Buy panty hose, opaque stockings, socks, and trouser socks in multiples. Scoop up at least six of each of your favorite shade of panty hose, like buff or barely black.

- Always buy a minimum of two pairs of patterned trouser socks. If one disappears in laundry sock cyberspace, you will still have a pair. Get in the habit of buying multiples in sport and workout socks. This is a super time-saver.

- House brands—brands created and manufactured by a store or chain—offer excellent value and style. Examples are INC in Federated stores such as Bloomingdale's and Macy's; Kate Hill in Lord & Taylor; Classiques Entier in Nordstrom; or simply clothing with the store name on the label. Such merchandise goes directly from manufacturer to the stores, cutting out the wholesale middleman and subsequent markup in price.

- Specialty shop clothing storeowners or managers usually know the best seamstress and tailor in their area and will be happy to recommend one.

- Move to a new city? Go to the city website and local a Newcomers group or neighborhood organization. Call and arrange to go to a meeting and steer conversation to favorite stores, shopping destinations, and services.

- Pick up and peruse weekly regional and neighborhood newspapers and magazines. They are filled with advertisements for small specialty boutiques and selective shops that can't afford to advertise in dailies. You may discover a favorite new shopping spot.

- Hair stylists are marvelous sources of shopping information. They're trained to be up on trends and interact with dozens of clients so they hear about new stores and new happenings in a community.

- During try-on times in the fitting room, always sit down, twist, and maybe even squat to make sure your choices—especially pants or jeans—will perform in your life.

- Make shopping for a swimsuit slightly less painful by applying a self-tanner lotion or cream the day or night before you set out for try-ons. You will look sun-kissed and svelte.

If you need us for questions or advice, visit us at www.optiondressing.com.

Judie and Jackie

INDEX

Page numbers in italics indicate box text.

A

A-line skirts, 146
AARP, 39
Abercrombie & Fitch, 64
Academy Awards, 40, 100
accessories, 158, 187–88
  body type and, 114
  Classic persona, 62
  with designer logos, 75,
    76, 202
  and focus, 208–09
  Modernist/Classic per-
    sona, 65
  Mood Dresser persona, 73
  organization of, 103–05
  outward expressions in,
    59
  packing, 232
  and self-esteem, 19
  shopping for, 236
  size and symmetry,
    194–98
  storage slots for, 103
  for travel, 221
  why you choose and wear
    them, 188–92
activities
  changing, 18
  clothing for, 3–6
  dictating wardrobe
    needs, 9
  in travel, 219
adaptation/adapters, 80–81

adolescents, 135–36
advertisements, 50, 168, 237
advice, 28
  about wardrobe, 22
age, 36, 77
  and body changes, 137
  and fashion persona, 77,
    78
  and Fashion Trend
    Trackers persona, 71
  issue of, 36–37, 38–39
  and pant style, 46
Age Venture News, 137
alterations, 98, 105, 122,
    128, 143
animal prints, 79
Anne Klein, 66
Anthropologie, 70
appearance
  and aura, 192
  changes, 55
  child, 27, 54
  dramatic, 77
  Dramatic Women per-
    sona, 75
  enhanced by accessories,
    187
  expression of psyche, 65
  feeling secure about, 28
  fixed beliefs about, 54
  judgments about, 22
  personality and, 60
  and society's valuation of
    women, 58

    sociocultural norms con-
      cerning, 136
    visual, 59
appearance signals, 214
appropriateness, 62
  handbag, 200–01
  hemlines, 123
  travel dress, 214, 217
April Cornell, 68
Arden B, 70
Armani, 66
arms, 122
artistic license, 73
artistic women, 74
athletic clothing/shoes, 79, 81
athletic gear, worn-out, 95
athletic persona, 68
  Natural persona, 63
attitude, 37–39
  projected by glasses,
    207–08
aura, 192
authentic self, 59, 61, 213

B

baby boomers, 137
backpacks, 211
balance
  accessories, 187–88
Banana Republic, 66
bargain shopping, 13, 15–16,
    39, 167

bargains, 13, 17, 167, 175
basic styles
    mix and match, 155
basics/basic pieces, 17
    at all price levels, 39
    "best friend," 16
    in geography change, 12
    in larger size, 10
    stocking up on, at sales,
      174, 175, 178
BCBG, 71
Bebe, 70, 78
bed covering, 87
behavior, 80
    changing, 74
    quirks of, 61
bell curve of fashion trends,
    80–81
belt buckle, 206, 207
belts, 120, 158, 204–07
    and body type, 114, 115
    storage, 103, 189
    for travel, 222
    wide, 114
Bergdorf's, 76
Bermuda shorts, 111
"best friend" clothes, 16
Betsey Johnson, 68
Better Homes and Gardens,
    38
Betts, Kate, 135
Big Boy ring, 193–94
Bill Blass, 63
Binchy, Maeve, 33–34
birth control pills, 136
black, 214, 232
black bottoms, 140
black clothes, 14, 46
black items
    marking, 107
black jacket, 159
black pants, 159
    buying, 169
black pantsuit, 181, 219
    for business event, 153, 154
black skirt, 143
black suit, 174
Blass, Bill, 70, 146
    see also Bill Blass

blazer, 12
    fashion personas, 61
Bloomingdales, 205, 237
blouses
    and body type, 114, 115
    in business dress, 157,
      158
    buyer and, 147
    draped, 117
    fashion personas, 67
    favorite, 130
    packing, 223
    tucked in, 111, 140
    as unit, 159
blouson, 120
body
    age and, 37
    balancing with acces-
      sories, 208–09
    clothes that fit, 174
    flawed, imperfect, 51–52
    insecurities about, 49
    preteen, 21
    shoes and, 205
    what works for, 28
body changes, 33, 136–37
body image, 49–50, 57, 109,
    134
    subjective, 135–36
Body Image Workbook
    (Cash), 49
body shapers, 129
body type(s), 113, 114–16,
    127
    and waistband, 139
bohemian women, 74
boots, 98, 204–05
boredom, 33
    shopping out of, 93, 165
bottoms
    basic color for, 225
    basic types, 148
    basics, 139–43
    building wardrobe from,
      133, 134, 138
    dress up from, 138–39
    favorite, 149
boys, outfitting, 68
brand name areas, 168

brand preferences, 170
bras, 231–32
    first, 136
    style, 129
breasts, 129, 136
    size, 115, 134
briefcases, 202, 218
Brockovich, Erin, 78
broomstick skirts, 145
Browns Boutiques, 200
browsing shopping day,
    233
browsing shops, 180
Buata, Mario, 188
Buchman, Dana, 63
budget, 21, 170
building blocks, 181
    skirts, 143–44
    of work wardrobe, 156
Burberry, 76
Bush, George W., 55
business, 1–18
    clothing styles in, 12
business cases, 202
Business Casual, 5, 11
    high side of, 151–63
    seminars defining guide-
      lines for, 153–54
Business Casual system,
    158–61
business dress, 151, 152, 153
    for business travel,
      220–21
    choice of, 158
    final analysis, 161–63
    hemlines, 123
    men/women difference,
      158
    new way of thinking
      about, 156–58
    relaxation of, 154–56
    short skirts and high
      heels with, 205
business travel/trips, 215,
    220–21, 222
    packing capsule for, 222,
      225–26
bust, 116
    large, 51, 115

bustline
  and jacket fit, 129
buttons, 128, 235
  missing, 222
buyers, 176
  pretending to be,
    146–48, 149
  and price points, 170–71

C

Cache, 78
California, 180
Calvin Klein, 66
camisoles, 117, 223
capri pants, 234
card case, 201
cardigan sweaters, 130, 157
career women, 18, 62, 155,
    156, 157
Carolina Herrera, 66
carpet in closet, 108
carry-on bag, 224
Cartier, 194
Cash, T. F., 49
Casual Fridays, 151–52, 155,
    157
casual wear
  for business trip, 220,
    221
  outfits, 171–72
  packing, 223
  skirts, 144
  tops, 101
  for travel, 222
catalog sales, 231
catalogs, 169, 181–83,
    233–34
  accessories in, 189
celebrities, imitating,
    166–67
cell phone, 201
CEO wives, 62
chain belts, 207
challenges, 31
  and cluttered closet, 93
Chanel, Coco, 29
change, 30, 34

desire for, 33
  personal calamities forc-
    ing, 31–32
chaos
  clearing, 91–108
charge accounts, 231
  list of numbers, 236
charity, 99, 105
  sorting things for, 98
Chaus, Josephine, 63
Chicago, 17, 214
childbirth, 137
child(ren)/childhood, 30
  appearance, 20
  body image, 135
  clothing budget, 21
  cruel taunts in, 53–54
  family's economic condi-
    tion in, 55–56
  feelings when shopping,
    20
  jewelry, 193
  teased about appearance,
    27, 54
China, 87
choices, 28, 30
chronological packers, 211,
    212
circle-cut skirts, 144
Circle of Friends (Binchy), 33
Circle of Life chart, 7*f*, 8
Circle of Life Game, 3–6
Circle of Your Life, 182
  redrawing, 18
circle scan, 172–73
cities, new, 33, 237
Classic/Dramatic fashion
    persona
  handbags, 199
Classic fashion persona, 19,
    61–63, 68, 78
  and fashion trends, 79,
    81
  finishing touches, *209*
  handbags, 199
  jewelry, 195, 196
Classic/Romantic fashion
    persona
  jewelry, 196

Classiques Entier, 237
cleaning out closet, 91
  feelings when, 25
  getting in mind-set,
    97–98
  organization blueprint,
    100–03
  payoff, 106–07
climate, 215, 228
clone dressing, 13–15
closet
  analyzing clothes in,
    171–72
  cluttered, 91–94
  as collection of life expe-
    riences, xv
  finances and size of,
    39–41
  full of clothes but noth-
    ing to wear, xv, 3
  ghosts from past in,
    51–54
  not in harmony with your
    life, 3, 8–9, 12
  learning in, 149
  "out-of-balance," 10–12
  personal layout, 101
  psychology of, xv, 18,
    42–58
  real you in, 3, 56–58
  reason for collecting
    goodies in, 94–95
  rethinking, 18
  revealing secrets, 44,
    45–46
  shopping in, 235
  sorting clothes in, 97–98,
    100–03
  suitcase as, 211–29
  system kits for, 102
  tips and tricks for setting
    up, 107–08
  unworn items in, 8
closet harmony, 9
Closet Insight Quiz, 96–97
closet makeovers, 32
closet space, expanding,
    101–02
closetology 101, 91–108

Clothes Diary, 15–17
    example, 16*f*
    sample, 18*f*
clothes/clothing, xv
    changes in, 74
    Classic persona, 61
    content and comfortable
        women, 28–29
    as costumes, 44–45
    with designer logos,
        75–76
    discarding while travel-
        ing, 228
    and emotional situations,
        34–35
    Fashion Trend Tracker
        persona, 69–70
    feelings about, as child, 20
    geographical roots in, 55
    getting rid of, 35
    hanging on body, 110–11,
        118
    Modernist persona, 65
    Mood Dresser persona,
        71–72
    Natural persona, 63
    never worn, 93, 99
    old, 95
    outward expressions in,
        59
    percent of, actually worn,
        8–9, 47
    projection of who you
        are, 44–45, 235
    as props for image and
        self-esteem, xv
    relationship with, 41
    rethinking, 18
    Romantic persona, 67
    selecting, 19–27
    and self-esteem, 19
    as self-expression, 28
    for travel activities, 219
    variance in types of, 57
clothes steamer, 228
clothing budget
    as child, 21
club meetings and lun-
    cheons, 6

coat(s), 12, 98, 177, 233
    ideal, 88
    travel, 219
cocktail look, 86, 146, 222
collars, 114, 117, 118, 181
college graduates, 62
color(s), 14, 17, 131, 140,
        176, 232–33
    arranging, 101
    belts, 206
    buy items in various, 101
    in catalogs and Internet
        sites, 182
    Dramatic Women per-
        sona, 75
    and fashion personas, 78
    fashion trends, 79
    handbags, 199
    mixing, 69
    personality and, 46
    power, 152
    short jackets, 128–29
    sportswear groups, 148
    stockings or trouser
        socks, 125
    travel wear, 214, 225–26
    variety, 85
comfort, 45
    for travel, 219
Comfort Boxes, 113–16
community activities
    hemlines, 123
    suits for, 157
company phone numbers,
    list of, 236
compartmentalizing packers,
    211, 212
competitive dressing, 214
compliments, 24, 27, 75
computer records, 149
concept(s), key
    in catalogs, 182
confidence, 27–28, 43, 58,
        163
    designer logos and, 75
    sense of, 19
    in social situations, 45
    in travel, 215
    your past and, 51–54

confidence issues, 30
confident but experimental
    women, 28
conflict issues, 167–69
connection, sense of, 58, 78
conservativeness, 29
    Classic persona, 61–63
consignment, 99, 105
    sorting things for, 98
consignment shop, 56, 93
    relationship with, 234
content and comfortable
    women, 28–29
contentment, 45
Corporate Casual, 151
corporate dress, 5, 154–55,
        157
    hemlines, 123
    relaxing, 11
    see also business dress
corporate wives, 40
cosmetic/beauty/fashion
    magazine industries, 50
cosmetics, 30
Cosmopolitan, 36, 38
costume jewelry, 196, 197
Covey, Stephen R., 213
co-workers
    judging your appearance,
        22
creativity, 74, 80
Cruise, Tom, 207–08
cultural dramatic dressers,
    77
cultural indicators
    in business, 161
Cummings, Angela, 70
customer service, 169
customers, 171
    classifying, 80

D

Dart, David, 139
date book, 15
daughters
    shopping, 63–64
Day, Doris, 56

Day-Timer, 15
de la Renta, Oscar, 188
   see also Oscar de la Renta
defects, 47
   women's magazines identifying, 50
Defining Details list, 158, *161*
Demko, David, 137
Denby, David, 50
department stores, 168, 169
   buyers, 149, 170–71
dependables, 16, 17
design refinement, 79
designer boutiques, 76
designer clothes, 39–40, 56
   hemlines, 123
   suits, 95
designer jewelry, 194, 197
designer label, 40, 41, 70
   and keeping clothes, 100
designer logos, 75–76, 87, 202
   on luggage, 218
designer merchandise
   distinguishing from knockoffs, 70
designers, 76, 81, 188
   hallmarks of work of, 70
   sarong-style wrap skirts, 145
   shoes, 204
   sportswear groups, 148
   use of elastic, 139
designs, 176
detail(s), 181, 187, 188
Details, 49
diamonds, 194
diets, 30
discount coupons/certificates, 175, 231
discount stores, 40, 62, 167, 203
DKNY, 66
Donna Karan, 66
double hanging, 101–02, 103
Dramatic fashion persona, 19, 74–78, 158
   and fashion trends, 79–80

finishing touches, *209*
   handbags, 199
   jewelry, 195, 196
   travel dress, 214
dress codes, 12, 214
"Dress for Success" era, 155
dress from bottoms up, 138–39
dresses, 143
   and body type, 114–15
   in business dress, 156
   buyer and, 147
   fashion persona, 67
   favorite, 130, 131
   packing, 223
   repeats, 235
   sorting, 101
   for travel, 227
   two-piece, 145
dressing
   factors in, 22
   from inside, xv, 128–29
dressing well, money in, 39
dressy occasion(s), 86
dressy skirts, 145–46
dressy something, 226–27
drop points, 108
dry cleaning, 98, 105
duffel bags, 211, *227*

E

early bird saving, 175
earrings, 67, 83, 187, 193, 195
   size of, 195
Eileen Fisher, 68
elastic waistbands, 139–40
   shorts, 142
Elie Tahari, 66
Elle, 69
emotional purchases, 16
emotional situations
   clothing and, 34–35
emotions, xv, 19, 32
   bargains and, 167
   closet as room of, 44
   and cluttered closet, 93, 94, 95

color and, 46
   Dramatic Women persona, 75
   evoked by clothes, 73
   and favorites, 130–32
   in handbags, 198
   in jewelry, 192
   and money, 39, 41
   with shoes, 204, 206
   shopping out of, 13
entrance makers, 75
Escada, 76
Esquire, 49
esteem issues, 34–35
   see also self-esteem
Europe, 214, 217
evening attire
   for travel, 220, 221, 222
evening bags, 202–03
events, packing for, *221*
exclusivity, 75
exercise clothes/gear, 9
   fashion personas, 63
   storage, 103–04
exotic ensembles, 73
experimenting, 28

F

fabrics, 40, 45, 70, 101, 181
   attention to, 236
   in business dress, 156–57
   and catalogs and Internet sites, 182
   Dramatic Women persona, 75
   fine, 56
   mixing, 69
   pleated pants, 126
   sheer and illusion-type, 232
   soft, 67
   solid, 85
   types of, 86
face
   accessories enhancing, 209
face shape, and glasses, 208

factory outlets, 235
fall clothes, 178
family, 1–18
    economic condition,
        55–56
fashion, 28
    fun in, 29
    secret code, 70
fashion chaos, 151
fashion cycles, 130, 177
    belts in, 206
    and interest in acces-
        sories, 188
    fashion jewelry, 196
    fashion magazines, 28,
        29, 30, 38
fashion persona(s), 29,
        59–90
    and accessories, 187
    and catalogs, 182
    combinations of, 78
    condensing, for travel,
        215
    discovering (quiz), 82–90
    and earrings, 195
    finishing touches, *209*
    in glasses, 208
    and handbags, 198–99
    and jewelry, 196
    minitrends, 81
    mixed, 199
    past, 106
    role of fashion trends in,
        79–80
    and shopping, 170
    split, 172
fashion personality(ies), 19, 56
    dominant, 60–78
fashion rules, 36
fashion season(s), 69, 233
fashion shows, 24, 29, 75,
        135, 177
fashion stars, 70
Fashion Trend Tracker fash-
        ion persona, 69–71, 75,
        78, 158
    and fashion trends,
        79–80, 81
    finishing touches, *209*

glasses, 208
    handbags, 199
fashion trends, 69, 111, 189
    bell curve of, 80–81
    jacket length, 128
    and jewelry, 196
    role in persona, 79–80
    sleeves, 122
Fast Company, 155
fat, 136
fathers, 52
favorites, 16, 17, 130–31
Fawcett, Farrah, 56
fear
    and memories in closet,
        94–95
feathers, 75
Federated stores, 237
feeling overwhelmed, 33
feelings about self, 18, 26
    clothes and, 43, 101,
        130–31
    shopping and, 13
feet, 203, 204, 209
figure problems, 35, 52
figure type
    and jeans, 141
    and pleats, 140
    see also body type(s)
Filofax, 15
finances
    and size of closet, 39–41
finishing touches, 187–209
    business dress, 158
Fisher, Eileen, 139
fit, 101, 138
    body proportions and, 111
    bottoms, 133
    in catalogs, 182
    jacket, 128–30
    shorts, 142
fitting room(s), 133–34, 238
fitting specialists, 235
flared skirts, 144
flashbacks, 54–56
Florida, 11, 73
    jewelry in, 197
    markdowns, 180–81
    Preview Season, 178

focal point, 187, 188
focus
    added by accessories,
        208–09
Fodors.com, 215
foot problems, 205–06
Forbes, 155
Ford, Tom, 140
Forever XXI, 70
Fragrance, 233, 235–36
frequent flyers, 228, 235
"Frequent Shopper" cards,
        231
friends
    comments from, 51
    judging your appearance,
        22
Friends, 56
full-length mirror, 47, 101,
        113, 124, 125, 127, 195,
        201, 234
    in closet, 108
fun, 1–18
Funny Feet Club, 188–89
fur, 75, 76

G

Gap, 64
Gentlemen Prefer Blondes
        (film), 196
geography, 11–12, 13–14,
        55, 77
    and fashion persona,
        78
    and jewelry, 197
gifts, 35, 86, 98, 104
    never worn, 57
Gill, Chris, 195–96
giving things away, 98–99
Glamour, 36, 138
glasses, 207–08
goals, wardrobe, 13
Golden Globes, 100, 166
gloves, 88
Good Housekeeping, 38
GQ, 49
grand tours, 215, 217

grooming aids
  packing, 223
group(s)
  mode of dress, 45
Gucci, 140
guilt
  in giving things away, 98
guilt inducers, 57, 99

H

hair/hairstyle, 28, 88, 158
  Dramatic Women per-
    sona, 75, 77
  media stars, 56
  new, 30
  Modernist persona, 66
  Natural persona, 63
  Romantic persona, 67
  upswept, 118
hair color, 235
hair stylists, 237
handbag parties, 199
handbags, 84, 187, 189
  buying guidelines,
    202–03
  with designer logos, 76
  Dramatic Women per-
    sona, 75
  Modernist persona, 66
  packing, 218, 223, 224
  self-expression in,
    198–203
  status, 81
  stolen, 236
  storage, 102, 103
  for travel, 222
hands, 209
hangers, 97
Hardy, John, 194
Harold's, 63
Harper's Bazaar, 36, 110, 203
Harrod's, 68
hassles, 169
hats
  Dramatic Women per-
    sona, 75
  storage, 103

head, accessories enhancing,
    209
heart thumpers, 176
height, 52, 128
help, needing, 30
Hemingway, Ernest, collec-
    tion, 79
hemlines, 36, 111
  pants, 125
Henri Bendel, 76
Hepburn, Audrey, 56, 110
high heels, 120, 204, 205
hip huggers, 46
hipbones, 110
hippies, 74
hips, 51, 136, 140
  wide, 142
Horizontal Line Dressing,
    112–32, 195
  moving lines to create
    flattering visual impres-
    sion, 116–32
hosiery, 87–88, 221
  buying in multiples, 237
  packing, 223
hot tips (list), 231–38
house brands, 237
husband
  needing approval from,
    25
  promoted, 33

I

"I don't have a thing to
  wear," xv, 3, 41
"I hate to shop" epidemic,
    167–69
ideal ensemble, searching
  for, 1–3
illness, 33
  life events and, 168–69
image issues, 29
  see also body image
impulse purchases, 12–13,
    15, 17
  Mood Dresser persona,
    71

In Style, 36, 69, 135
inability to throw anything
  away, 55
INC, 71, 237
inflation, 171
inner self
  watches and, 197–98
insecurity(ies), 54
  clothes overcoming, 45
  mirror and, 47–50
  in travel, 213–14
inside
  dressing from, xv, 128–29
  person on, 59
insider secrets (list), 231–38
instant gratification, 183,
    189
intentions not materialized,
    9
interests, 37–39
  expressed in jewelry,
    193
  indicated by logos, 202
interlocker packers, 211,
    212
Internet, 37
  accessories, 189
  shopping on, 181–83
  shopping sites on, 170
inverted triangle, 125, 143
Italy, 228–29

J

J. Crew, 64
jacket(s), 85
  and body type, 114, 115
  bright, over dark sepa-
    rates, 234
  in business dress, 156,
    157, 158
  buyer and, 147, 148
  fashion personas, 65
  favorites, 130, 131
  feelings about wearing,
    26
  fit, 128–30
  heavy, 98

jacket(s) (cont.)
  packing, 223
  red, 152
  sleeves, 121
  sorting, 101
  "stand alone," 226
  as unit, 159
jacket length/shape, 116,
  126–30
  and hemlines, 123
Jane (magazine), 36, 138
jeans, 46, 134, 222
  basic item, 141–42
  fashion personas, 63, 65
  that fit, 138, 232
  shopping for, 232
Jeffrey, 70
Jessica McClintock, 68
jewelry, 83, 158, 187, 192–94
  cost and selection,
    195–97
  designer, 70
  Dramatic Women per-
    sona, 75
  Modernist persona, 66
  Mood Dresser persona,
    73
  Romantic persona, 67
  sizes, 195
  storage, 104–05, 189
  for travel, 221, 222
  see also necklaces
job changes, 11, 12
"job interview closet," 93
Jones New York, 66, 148, 168

K

Karan, Donna, 145
Kate Hill, 237
Keaton, Diane, 56
Kelly, Grace, 56
key cases, 202
khaki pants/shorts, 63, 156,
  157
Kidman, Nicole, 166
knit pants, 156
knit tops, 157, 222

buyer and, 148
favorite, 130
horizontal stripes on, 119
knits, 219
  folded, 102, 103
  sorting, 101
knockoffs, 40, 70, 76
  handbags, 199
  watches, 198
Kohn, Lafreniere, and
    Gutevich
  research team, 169
Krantz, Judith, 181

L

L.L. Bean, 64
Ladies' Home Journal, 36
"ladies who lunch," 62
Lagos, 194
laser shoppers, 170
  keys to becoming, 180
Lauren, Ralph, 66, 72
  see also Ralph Lauren
Lauren by Ralph Lauren, 66
layering, 228
layering in, 120
leather, 76
  belts, 206, 207
  handbags, 202–03
leg length, 110, 115, 127, 128
  and shorts, 143
Legally Blonde (film), 50
legs, 51, 52
  long, 120
  and short skirts, 144
leisure activities, clothes for,
  8–9
life
  circle of, 1–18
  rethinking, 18
life changes/transitions,
  10–12, 18
  clothes markers of, 57
  and fashion persona, 78
  and fear of loss, 94
life events
  jewelry marking, 193

in stress and illness,
  168–69
life history
  clothes reveal, 56
  and who you are today, 58
life "makeover," 32
life role(s), passages
  between, 32
life stages, 36–37
lifestyle
  and body change, 136
  new, 12
  and shopping, 170
lighting in closets, 102–03
Lillie Rubin, 78
lingerie, 84, 221
  packing, 223
  for travel, 222, 223
little black dress (LBD), 29,
  227
Liz Claiborne, 148, 168
loafers, 61
logo ladies, 75–76, 81
logos
  on handbags, 202
  see also Designer logos
long over narrow look, 120
long over short rule, 120
long-waisted, 111, 113, 114,
  115, 120
look(s), 43–44
  experimenting with dif-
    ferent, 73–74
  of Modernist persona, 66
  new, 32
"look of the season," 79
Lord & Taylor, 68, 237
Loren, Sophia, 232
Los Angeles, 214
loss, fear of, 94
love(s)
  and feeling inadequate
    about dressing, 22
luggage, 213
  lifting, 217
  lost, 214, 224
  wheeled, 217–18
Lycra, 129, 219, 232
Lynne, Lori, 196

M

Macy's, 205, 237
Mademoiselle, 36, 38
magazines, 39, 138
  fashion trends in, 80
  male models in, 49
  regional and neighbor-
    hood, 237
  women's defects in, 50
  women's relationship to,
    37–38
  see also fashion maga-
    zines; women's maga-
    zines
makeovers, 30, 32, 33, 77
makeup, 30, 83, 158, 235
  Dramatic Women per-
    sona, 75, 77
  Modernist persona, 66
  Natural persona, 63
mall(s), 62, 70
  expeditionary mission to,
    148–49
Marc Jacobs, 71
Marie Claire, 36, 203
markdown mistakes, 99–100
markdowns, 167, 175, 176,
    180, 231
  in Florida, 181
match-up piece(s), 175
Max Mara, 66
Max Studio, 70
media, 48
  size issue in, 49
  women's relationship to,
    37
media stars, imitating, 56,
    166–67
medications
  and body change, 136
memories in closet
  fear, potential, and
    94–95
men
  business cases, 202
  and Business Casual, 152,
    154, 155
  business dress, 158

closets, 102
  percent of clothes worn,
    47
  phobia about shopping,
    165
  wedding ring, 193
menopause, 137
merchandise display, 169
Michael Kors, 71
minitrends, 81
miniwardrobes
  in different sizes, 57
mirrors, 21, 34, 109, 136, 140
  and insecurities, 47–50
  three-way, 128, 142
  see also full-length mir-
    ror
misses sizes, 173–74
mistakes, 16, 17, 34
  making over and over, 9
  markdown, 99–100
  in packing suitcase,
    213–14
  selling, 234
mixing and matching, 57, 64,
    146, 147, 149, 222
  basic styles, 155
models
  in catalogs, 181–82
  male, 49–50
  pegged skirts, 124
  shorts, 142
  skinny, 135
Modern Maturity, 38
Modernist/Classic fashion
    persona, 65
Modernist fashion persona,
    64–66, 78, 172
  and fashion trends, 80
  finishing touches, *209*
  handbags, 199
  jewelry, 196
money, 100
  relationship with, 39–41
  spending, 165
  wasted, 99
Monroe, Marilyn, 196
Mood Dresser fashion per-
    sona, 57, 71–74, 158

and fashion trends, 80
  finishing touches, *209*
  glasses, 208
  handbags, 199
  jewelry, 195
More magazine, 38
Morris, Robert Lee, 70
Moss, Kate, 135
mother/daughter dressing,
    68
mothers, messages from,
    51–53
motivations, 15, 32–33
  in buying and returning
    clothes, 179–80
  for makeovers from pro-
    fessionals, 32
  in shopping, 47, 165, 185
moving, 11–12, 33, 237
MTV, 38, 69
  fashion shows, 24
  influence of, 56
multiples, 138
  hosiery, 237
  shorts, 143
muscle mass, 137
must-have status, 81
My Generation, 38

N

nail polish, 83–84
Native American handi-
    crafts, 197
Natural fashion persona,
    63–64, 172
  and fashion trends, 79,
    81
  finishing touches, *209*
  glasses, 208
  handbags, 199
  jewelry, 195, 196
neck, 110, 117–18
  camouflaging, 232
  long, 195
necklaces, 118, 187, 195
  long, 117, 232
  storage, 103, 189

neckline, 117–19, 131
  jacket, 128
  and sleeve length, 122
neckties, 152, 154
negative attitudes toward
    yourself, 40, 54–55
Neiman Marcus, 76
new classic(s), 79
new job, 33
  and fashion persona, 78
  see also job change
new man, 33
New York City, 12, 46, 172,
    199, 213–14
  shoes, 204, 205
New Yorker, The, 50
newspapers, regional and
    neighborhood, 237
Nicole Miller, 66
Nike, 137
Nordstrom, 63, 237
nostalgia box, 104–05
nostalgia corner, 99–100
Nygard, Peter, 139

O

O, The Oprah Magazine, 38
obsession, 30
"one-look dressing," 14
order, establishing, 91–108
organization, 56–57, 73
  of accessories, 103–05
organization blueprint,
    100–03
Oscar de la Renta, 68, 70
out-of-season clothes, 97, 98
outerwear, 158
outfits, 70, 147, 160
  Dramatic Women per-
    sona, 75
  favorite, 66, 100, 107
  hanging together, 56–57
  jacket in, 126
  new combinations for, 106
  putting together, 23, 28,
    146
  shoes and, 205

skirt length and, 234
sportswear groups,
    148–49
for travel, 219, 221, 222
trying on, 43
units and, 159–61
outlet directories, 236
outlet stores, 177

P

packing, 222
  dress rehearsal, 222–23
  in layers, 222, 223–24
  mistakes in, 213–14
  for wedding, graduation,
    or christening, *221*
  for weekend getaway,
    227
  what goes where, 223–24
packing capsule
  for business trips,
    225–26, 229
packing pyramid, 220–22
packing tips, 228–29
pajamas, 6
Palm Beach, 214
Paltrow, Gwyneth, 56
pant legs, 111, 126
pant length, 111, 116,
    125–26
pant style
  and age, 46
pants, 12, 143
  basic item, 139–41
  in business dress, 156,
    157
  buyer and, 147, 148
  casual, for travel, 227
  cuffs, 125–26
  fashion personas, 65
  favorite, 130, 131, 149
  that fit, 138–39
  hangers for, 97
  narrow, 120
  packing, 223
  pleated/flat-front, 46, 79,
    126, 140–41, 234

pockets on, 141
  sorting, 101
  stretched-out, 95
  as unit, 159
pantsuits, 52, 65, 142
  in business dress, 152,
    158
  for travel, 219
parents, messages from,
    51–53
Parton, Dolly, 55
past (the), 77
  and confidence, 51–54
  influence of, in Romantic
    persona, 67
  looking back to, 54–56
pastel colors, 67
Patagonia, 64
pattern choice, 141
patterns, 85, 86
  scarves, 191–92
pearls, 117, 158, 193
  fashion personas, 67
peasant dressing, 80
pegging skirts, 123–24
pendant drops, 117
People magazine, 49, 208
perceived value, 170, 183
perception, xv
  change in, 34
  of self, 51, 54
  shoes and, 205
perfumes, 233
Perretti, Elsa, 70, 207
persona, 59
  see also fashion persona(s)
Persona Pieces list, 158, 161,
    161
personal calamities
  forcing change, 31–32
personal growth
  transitions and, 32–34
personal issues, 33
personal shoppers, 30, 235
personal style, 19
  and varying your
    wardrobe, 15
personalities, multiple, 72,
    73

personality
    and appearance, 59–60
    clothes reflecting, 47
    expression of, 213
    fragrance and, 233
    handbags and, 198
    indicated by logos, 202
    items in closet revealing,
        46
petite department, 115
petites, 115, 126, 173
    and accessories, 195
    jacket length, 127–28
phone numbers, list of, 236
physical fitness revolution,
    37
piano shawl, 192
picture(s), 21
    old, 54–55
pin(s), 187, 195, 196
pivotal pieces, 126–27
    for travel, 226–27
plan, 17–18
plastic bags for packing,
    223–24
pleasure travel, 215
pleats
    in pants, 46, 126,
        140–41, 234
    in shorts, 143
    in skirts, 146
Polartec, 63
polo shirts, 46
pop stars, 166
potential
    and memories in closet,
        94–95
power suits, 152, 163
Prada, 71
pregnancy, 136–37
preseason sale time, 178
preseason shopping, 166
Preview Season, 178
price points, 170–71, 183
Prince of Tides (film), 166–67
prints
    mixing, 69
    small, 67
private sales, 231

professional advice, 31–32
Professional Casual, 161–63
proportion illusions, stripes
    in, 234
proportion(s), 29, 109–32,
    140, 170, 172, 173
    and belts, 207
    exercise, 130–32
    in jewelry, 195
    shorts and, 142
psyche, 99, 109, 165
    appearance expressing,
        65
    jewelry and, 104
    self-presentation in, xv
    what works for, 28
psychic disfigurement, 54
psychographics, 37–39
psychology of closet, xv, 18,
    42–58
puberty, 135–36
pull-on pants, 46
pumps, plain, 61
punch pieces, 187–209

R

raincoats, 98
Ralph Lauren, 68, 76, 148,
    168
Ray Ban Aviators, 208
Ray Ban Wayfarers, 207–08
Real Simple, 38
real you
    unveiling, in closet,
        56–58
rebuying the same thing, 98
red
    power color, 152
Redbook, 36
Redford, Robert, 55
refund specifications, 179
regional American looks, 73
relationship changes, 33
repair (clothes), 98–99, 101
repeats, 65, 80, 235
replacement(s), 101, 107,
    165, 222, 234

Modernist persona, 66
    tops, 101
resort collections, 233
retail therapy, 165, 181
return policies, 178–80
return to store for credit, 93
returns
    mail order and Internet
        orders, 183
risk takers, 69, 79
Risky Business (film), 207
Roberts, Julia, 56, 78, 100
roller packers, 211, 212
romance, 1–18
Romantic fashion persona,
    19, 67–68
    and fashion trends,
        80–81
    finishing touches, *209*
    jewelry, 195
ruffles, 67
Russell, Jane, 196

S

St. John, 76, 139
St. John Knits, 63
Saks, 76, 205
sale rack philosophy and
    success, 174–76
sale tips, 176
sales, 13, 14, 40, 167, 231
sales associate, 14, 169, 236
sales clerks, 17
sales receipt, 179
San Francisco, 11–12, 180
sarong-style skirts, 124,
    144–45, 234
Savvy Department at
    Nordstrom, 70
scale, 24
    accessories, 187–88
Scandinavia, 214
scarves, 158, 191–92
    storage, 104, 189
    for travel, 222, 227
seamstresses, 237
seasonal bonanzas, 180–81

seasonal fashion calendars, 177–78
seasonal sales, 235
seasons, clothes for, 98
secrets
    closet revealing, 45–46
"security blankets," 100
selecting clothes
    self-discovery quiz, 19–30
self (the), 28
    authentic, 59, 61
    real/ideal, 74
self-concept, 136
    body image in, 135
self-confidence, xv, 44, 134, 202
self-definition, 19–41, 57
self-discovery, 32
    quiz, 19–30
self-esteem, 19, 27, 30, 34–35, 43, 125
    daily search for, 44–45
    designer logos and, 75
    money and, 39–40
    and wardrobe size, 41
self-exploration, 170
self-expression, 74
    clothes as, 28
    in handbag, 198–203
    internal, 59–90
    in travel dress, 214
self-image, 19, 28
    body change and, 137
    different from what world sees, 33–34
    and fashion persona, 78
    the vamp, 77
self-improvement, 30
self-knowledge, xv, 31–32, 180
self-monitor
    Classic persona, 62
    Dramatic Women persona, 75
    Natural persona, 64
self-presentation, xv
sense of dress, 23
sense of self, 27
    body in, 136

sense of style, 28, 60, 147
separates, 145–46, 175, 234
separation anxiety, 35, 98–99
Seventeen, 36, 53
Sex and the City, 38
sexy persona, 52, 77–78
shawls, 227, 232
    Dramatic Women persona, 75
shelf (closet), 102, 103
Shelli Segal for Laundry, 71
shipping charges, 182–83
shirts, 148
    big/oversize, 130
    tailored, 61, 63
shoe size, 188–89, 206
shoes, 125, 187, 199–200, 203–06, 209
    business dress, 82, 158
    Dramatic Women persona, 75
    for evening, 82
    fashion personas, 65, 67
    outdated, 95
    packing, 224
    saving, 196
    storage slots for, 103
    for travel, 219, 221, 222, 228
shopping, 34, 133–34, 165–85
    alone or with friends, 25
    Classic persona, 62, 63
    in closet, 106–07, 235
    confident but experimental women, 28
    content and comfortable women, 29
    with daughters, 63–64
    Dramatic Women persona, 76, 78
    dressing for, 233
    Fashion Trend Tracker persona, 69–71
    on Internet, 81–83
    for jeans, 232
    Modernist persona, 66

Mood Dresser persona, 74
Natural persona, 63, 64
    purpose and direction in, 172, 180
    quiz, 183–85
    reasons for, 47, 165–66
    Romantic persona, 68
    for spring, 177–78
    as substitute for what is really wanted in life, 93
    superconfident women, 27–28
    for swimsuit, 238
    while traveling, 228, 236
    on vacation, 24, 62
shopping emporiums, dysfunctional
    attacking, 169–73
shopping habits, 9
    pattern in, 183–85
    poor, 12–13
shopping list, 3, 17, 101, 107, 171, 180
shopping patterns, changes in, 15
shopping trips
    group, 176
    planning, 180
short skirts, 144, 146
short-waisted, 111, 113, 114, 115, 120, 121, 127
    and belts, 207
    and shorts, 143
shorts, 133
    basic item, 138, 142–43
    buyer and, 147, 148
shoulder line, 117–19, 128
shoulder pads, 118–19
shoulder width, 118–19
shoulders, bare, 117
signature style, 64
Silicon Valley, 151, 152, 161
silk blouses, 65
silverware, 87
simplicity, 64
situational persona, 61
size, 49, 170, 173–74
    and accessories, 194–98

Americans increasing in, 137
issues about, 49
labeled incorrectly, 176
miniwardrobes in different, 57
overestimating, 135
unhappiness with, 23
size charts, 182, 234
size designations, 137
size ranges, 173–74
size reality, disparity in, 135
skimming and slimming skirts, 144
skirt length, 116, 123–25
ankle, 124
and outfits, 234
skirts, 12, 65, 101, 133
ankle-length, 124
basic item, 138
in business dress, 156, 157
buyer and, 147, 148
fashion personas, 61, 67
favorite, 130, 131, 149
hangers for, 97
long slim, 120
midcalf length, 124
packing, 223
pegged, 123–24
right style, 143–46
slits, 123
sorting, 101
as unit, 159
without waistbands, 121
sleepwear, 6, 84
packing, 222, 223
sleeve length, 121–22
sleeveless dresses, 36
sleeves, 111, 121
social attitude, 48
social events
needing approval for outfits at, 25
social life, 9
social situations
confidence in, 45
judging your look by what others are wearing, 23

society
valuation of women, 58
sofa, 88
soft dressing, 219
someday clothes, 9–10, 11, 15, 99–100
soul-searching, 33
South, jewelry in, 197
Southwest, 14, 73, 77, 145
jewelry in, 197
Spade, Kate, 81
spandex, 129
special event dressing, 220, 221, 222
special events, clothes markers of, 59
specialty stores, 62, 138, 173, 235, 237
spending limit, 171
Sports Unlimited, 64
sportswear, 168, 172
in catalogs, 181
fashion personas, 63
sportswear groups, 148–49
repeats of, 235
"stall" mode, 32
status, 76, 80, 81
step stool, 108
stiletto heels, 204–05
stockings, 125
see also hosiery
stole, 232
storage
"story" pieces, 100
underbed, 108
storage boxes, 98, 102
storage organizers, 103
store layouts, 170
store racks, 169, 173
store specialist(s), 235
stores
circle scan, 172–73
designer departments, 71
dressing rooms, 109
fashion trends in, 80
out-of-town, 235
specialized, 14
walking tour through, 235

"story" pieces, 99–100
Storybook Heirlooms catalog, 68
Streisand, Barbra, 27, 167
stress, 32, 33, 37
life events and, 168–69
stripes, 119, 141
proportion illusions, 234
stud earrings, 67
style(s), 17, 176
duplicating basics in, 101
evolution in, 158
finding at sales, 174
tracking favorite, 149
subconscious, 50
price points in, 170
suits, 70, 101, 106, 157
for business, 154, 155, 158
buyer and, 147
fashion personas, 61
designer, 70
Modernist persona, 65
as outfit, 159
power, 163
splitting into separate pieces, 11, 145–46, 156
suitcase
as closet, 211–29
packing, 211–12, 223–24
packing mistakes, 213–14
suitcase simplification, five *W*s of, 216
summer clothes, 178
Sunbelt, 122, 177, 180, 233
sundresses, 117
super bargains, 12–13, 16, 167
superconfident women, 27–28
"survival gear," packing, 224
survival gear options, 224–25
swap parties, 98, 106
sweater sets, 11, 157, 174, 219
sweaters, 45, 85, 157
buyer and, 148
fashion personas, 65
horizontal stripes on, 119

sweaters *(cont.)*
   packing, 223
   with short skirts, 144
   with skirts, 146
   sorting, 101
   storage, 103, 108
swimsuits, 25, 50, 87, 111,
   134, 178
   and body type, 115
   on sale, 177
   shopping for, 238
   storage, 103
symmetry
   accessories, 194–98

T

tailored shirts, 61, 63
tailors, 237
Talbots, 63
tall sizes, 111, 173, 174
tank tops, 117
Target, 71
tees, 46
   in business dress, 156
   buyer and, 148
   cotton, 174
   fashion personas, 63, 65
   knit, 222
   packing, 223
   with short skirts, 144
   storage, 103
television, 37, 38
   fashion trends on, 80
Texas, 145
Texas Head Turners, 77
textures, 70
   mixing, 69, 128
therapy, shopping as, 167
   see also retail therapy
thighs, 51, 126
thinness, obsession with, 135
Thompson, J. Kevin, 49, 135
thong panties, 140
Title Nine Sports, 64
"to do" list, 101
Tommy Hilfiger, 64, 148, 168
Top Gun (film), 208

tops, 133
   basic, 148
   and body type, 115
   in business dress, 156, 157
   buyer and, 147, 148
   colors, 225
   halter-style, 119
   one-shouldered, 234
   packing, 223
   for short-waisted women,
     121
   sleeves, 121
   sorting, 101
   tight, 134, 135
   tuckers/nontuckers, 120
   see also knit tops
tote bag(s), 218, 224
Tracy, Ellen, 63
training seminars
   Business Casual guide-
     lines, 153–54
transitions
   and personal growth,
     32–34
travel stops, 180–81
Travelsmith.com, 227
traveling, 30, 211–29
   with as little as possible,
     217
   master plan, 215
   packing mistakes, 213–14
   pivotal pieces, 226–27
   shopping, 228, 236
   starting with basics,
     217–19
   written itinerary, 218–19,
     222
trend reruns, 180–81
trendy clothes, 176
trouser socks, 158, 237
   color, 125
   fashion personas, 61
trousers, 125, 133
   base item, 138
   fashion personas, 61
Trump, Blaine, 39
trumpet skirt, 144
trunk shows, 75
try-on, 101, 234, 238

tummy, 140, 141, 143
turtlenecks, 111, 117, 157
"Tyranny of Skinny, The,
   Fashion's Insider Secret"
   (Betts), 135

U

umbrellas, 98
unconstructed jackets, 129
units, 159–61
University of South Florida,
   49
US magazine, 49

V

vacations, 215
   buying accessories on,
     189
   packing for, 221–22
   shopping on, 24, 62
   skirts for, 144
   travel itinerary, 222
Valentino, 63, 100
vamp, the, 77–78
Vanity Fair, 197, 203
vanity sizing, 137
Vass, Joan, 139
Versace, 76
versatility, 158
   pivotal pieces add,
     226–27
   travel dress, 219
vertical lines, 116, 119, 121
vests, 115
vintage clothing, 68, 69, 190
vintage designer clothes,
   100
visual illusions, 112, 122, 144
   with belts, 207
visual impression, flattering,
   116–32
Vogue, 36, 49, 110, 203
Von Furstenberg, Diane, 181
VPL (visible panty line), 140
Vreeland, Diana, 110

W

waist, 115–16
  and belts, 207
  fitted, 114
  position of, 110, 113
  and shorts, 143
waistline, 111, 115, 116,
    119–21, 136
  pleats at, 140
  weight below, 126, 127
waistbands, 120, 139–40
  shorts, 143
walk-in closets, 103
Wall Street Journal, 155
wallets, 201–02
  stolen, 236
Wal-Mart, 71
Wang, Vera, 223
wardrobe
  activities dictating, 9
  asking for advice about, 22
  building, 133–49
  buying additions, 235
  creating, 23
  editing, 30
  feelings about, 34
  lifestyle, 12
  parts missing, 3
  putting together, 28
  rethinking, 12
  in sync with life, 3, 9, 18
  varying, 15
  for work, 154–56

wardrobe makeovers, 32
wardrobe "tune-up," 30
watchband, 88
watches, 197–98
weather
  and travel, 213, 215
Web catalog clicks, 12–13
weekend getaway, packing
    for, *227*
weekend wear, 123, 153, 215
weeklong vacations, 215
weight, 52, 57, 137
  below waistline, 126, 127
weight changes, 10–11, 32,
    33, 101
  and pant length, 126
  and proportions, 110
Wet Seal, 70
wheelies, *221*
white shoes, 36
who you are
  expressed in jewelry,
    193
  today, 58
window-shopping, 70
women
  "stuck in time," 77
  work categories, 155
  work in progress, 29–30,
    33
women who work outside
    the home, 62
women's magazines, 36–38
  swimsuit issues, 50

see also fashion maga-
    zines
women's sizes, 173, 174
wooden pegs, hooks, 108
work, 8
  dressing for, 4, 5–6
  at home, 5–6
work clothes, 5, 154–56, 171
  arranging, 101
  unworn, 8
work in progress women,
    29–30, 33
working out, dressing for, 6
wrap(s), 117
  for travel, 227
wrap dresses, 234
wrap skirts, 124, 144–45
wrist line, 116, 121–22
wrists, 209

Y

Yankelovich Monitor survey,
    169
Yellow Pages, 235
Yesterdaze, 173
YM (Young Miss), 36, 138
Yurman, David, 70, 194

Z

Zellweger, Renée, 49, 100

ABOUT THE AUTHORS

JUDIE TAGGART is a fashion professional with more than two decades of experience in retailing as a designer buyer, an advertising executive, and the fashion director of three retail department store chains. During this period and in later work in marketing and the media, Judie learned the power of clothes to transform a woman's image of herself and alter her emotional viewpoint. Helping women understand this concept and how to do it in a positive, supportive way is a recurrent theme in her writings and in this book.

As the fashion editor of *The Tampa Tribune* for six years, she became a fashion critic "looking from the outside in." As a fashion editor and also a correspondent for Fairchild News Service, Judie covered the fashion collections, interviewed designers, and reported on breaking trends in New York, California, and the world. Her writing has appeared in *Women's Wear Daily, W, Cosmopolitan, The Tampa Tribune,* and *The San Francisco Chronicle,* among others.

Currently Judie has her own firm, Taggart and Company, a retail consultancy. She speaks to convention groups on lifestyle issues for executive and professional women, and appears on local television interview and news programs.

JACKIE WALKER'S career spans more than twenty-five years in the fashion retail industry and the human resources field. Fashion showed her the importance of creating an image on the outside, but human resources taught her that success must start from within. Blending these became her mission.

In 1988 Jackie created Option Dressing, a company designed to help people discover who they are on the inside and learn how that relates to what they wear each day. Jackie has worked with hundreds of individuals, including politicians, media personalities, and top CEOs. Her success led to the creation of a series of motivational and informational workshops and training sessions based on her philosophy, and these local and regional appearances earned her the title the "Dr. of Closetology."

Jackie is a monthly fashion contributor on FOX 13 TV's *Good Day Tampa Bay.* She is also a featured keynote and workshop speaker for Southern Women's Shows, Inc., and for women's conferences and expos across the nation.